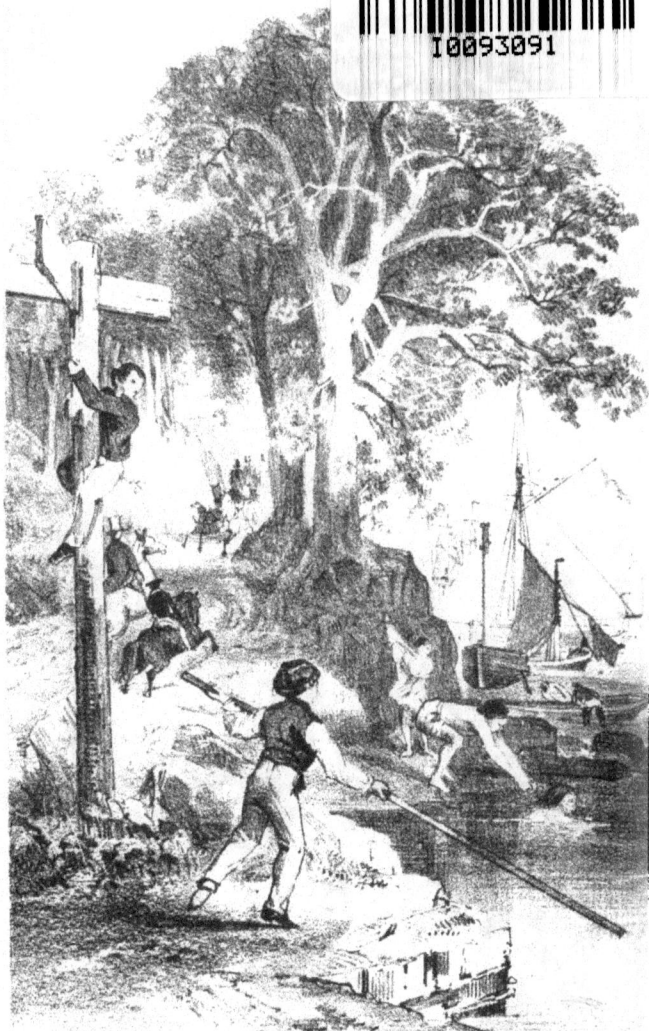

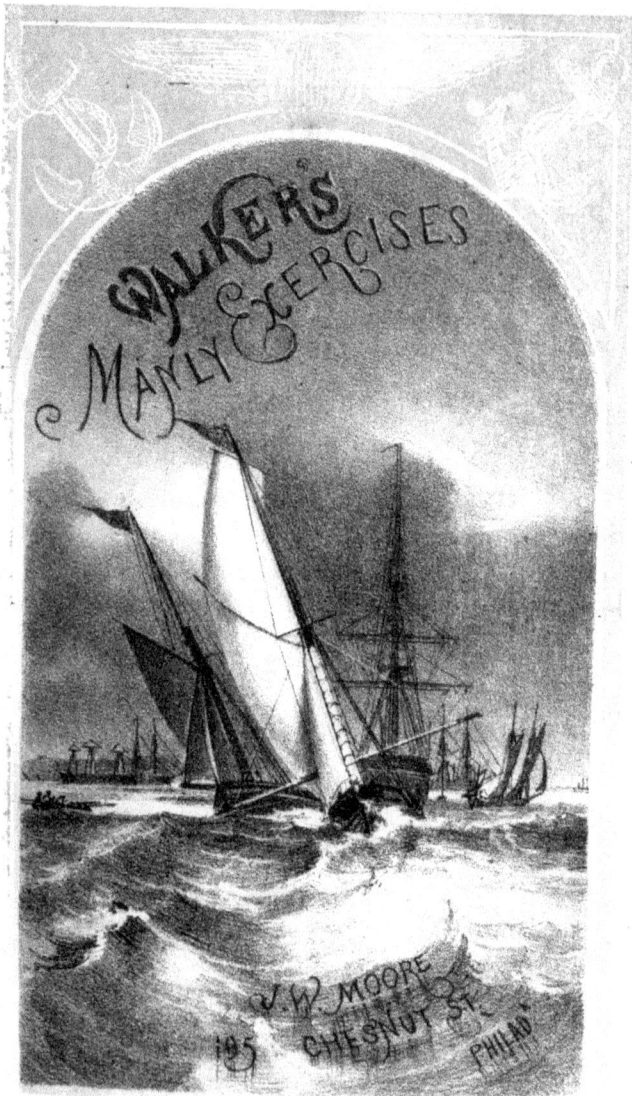

Printed by Wagner & McGuigan, Phil:

WALKER'S

MANLY EXERCISES;

CONTAINING

Rowing, Sailing, Riding, Driving, Racing, Hunting, Shooting,

AND OTHER MANLY SPORTS.

THE WHOLE CAREFULLY REVISED OR WRITTEN,

By "CRAVEN."

FROM THE NINTH LONDON EDITION.

PHILADELPHIA:
PUBLISHED BY JOHN W. MOORE
NO. 195 CHESTNUT STREET.
1856.

PRINTED BY HENRY B. ASHMEAD.

GEORGE ST. ABOVE ELEVENTH.

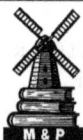

EDITOR'S PREFACE.

THE publishers of the present Edition of this popular little volume had a double purpose in entering upon the undertaking,—namely, to offer a carefully-revised copy of *Walker's Manly Exercises*, and an outline of *Rural Sports*, to which they serve as the best elementary introduction. As the execution of that design was committed to me, I can only allude to the nature of the task, and hope that I have not quite failed in the enterprise. This I *may* be permitted to say,—that if the publisher's desire to make the work a source of instructive and rational amusement be realized, even to the tithe of its extent and earnestness, the labor of his Editor will not have been wholly without success.

CRAVEN.

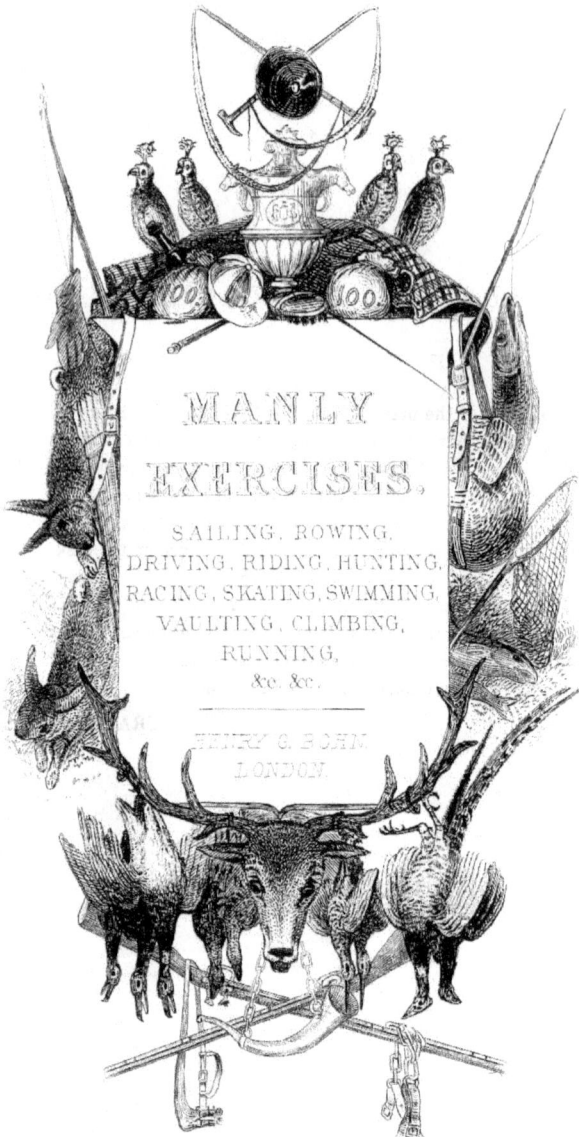

MANLY EXERCISES.

SAILING. ROWING.
DRIVING. RIDING. HUNTING,
RACING, SKATING, SWIMMING,
VAULTING, CLIMBING,
RUNNING,
&c. &c.

HENRY G. BOHN.
LONDON.

CONTENTS.

IMPORTANCE OF PHYSICAL EXERCISES.

LOCOMOTIVE EXERCISES.

1*

AQUATIC EXERCISES.

RIDING.

CONTENTS.

LIST OF PLATES.

FRONTISPIECE.

Vignette.

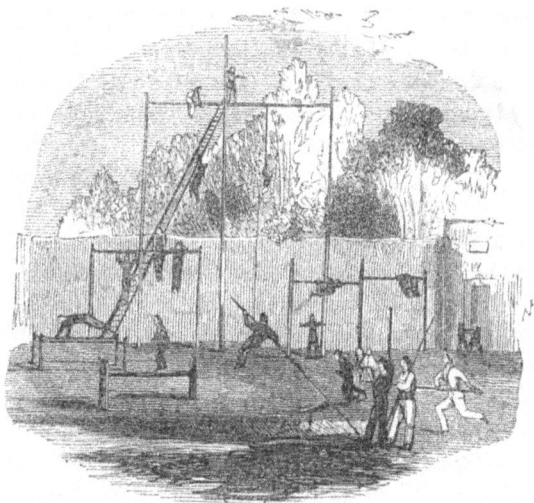

IMPORTANCE OF PHYSICAL EXERCISES.

EDUCATION may be divided into two parts, physical and mental. Of the former, EXERCISES or GYMNASTICS are the most extensive and the earliest portion.

THEIR EXTENT is learnt by an enumeration of them, viz., Walking, Running, Leaping, Vaulting, Pole-leaping, Balancing, Skating, Carrying, Climbing, and Swimming. We have added Throwing the Discus; and, in a course of British Exercises, we think Rowing, Sailing, Riding, and Driving, would be very improperly omitted.

The object of these Exercises is to strengthen the muscular system, by subjecting it to a regular process of training, and to teach the means of employing it most advantageously. The expediency of their early acquisition

2

is rendered evident by the first tendency of youth being directed to them, by the rapid progress made in them, and by the delight derived from them, at a period when the body is incapable, with real or solid advantage, of higher acquirements.

Their general utility will be questioned only by those who are not aware that the health and vigor of all the bodily organs depend on the proportioned exercise of each. In active exertion, the member exercised swells with the more frequent and more copious flow of blood, and heat is developed in it with greater abundance; and if we repeat the same motions many times after intervals of repose, all the muscles exercised become permanently developed; a perfection of action ensues in the member exercised, which it did not previously possess, any deformity by which it is affected is corrected, and strength and activity are acquired. That man, therefore, gains the most strength who engages in muscular exercises that require the application of much power, but which are sufficiently separated by intervals of repose.

It must be remembered, however, that, in exercising particular muscles only, the others become weak. The strength of Marshal Saxe was sufficiently great to stop a chariot drawn at speed by four horses, by merely seizing the wheel: he bent pieces of silver with his fingers, made them into boats as he would with paper, and presented them to the ladies. Count Orloff, a Russian general, broke the shoe of a carriage horse in the same manner; and there are innumerable examples of similar feats of extraordinary strength.

Active exercises, at the same time, confer beauty of form; and they even contribute to impart an elegant air and graceful manners. If the exercise of a limb be continued for some time, the member swells, a painful sensation is experienced, which is termed lassitude, and a difficulty of contraction, which is the result of it. If the motion has been excessive, and the organic elements in the member have been acted upon beyond all physiological laws, inflammation would take place, and its functions be performed with great difficulty, if at all.

Such are the effects of exercise on the locomotive system, to all the functions of animated beings, so long as they are exercised with moderation, equality, and at due intervals, working for their own preservation. Of course, the general effect of active exercises is marked in proportion to the number of parts that share in the motion, or are brought into energetic action. In general exercise, the increase of organic action is not confined solely to the parts which are the seat of muscular contraction, but is repeated throughout all parts of the economy, and influences all the functions.

Thus, as to the vital or nutritive system, exercises taken when digestion is not going on, excite the digestive faculty: taken during its progress, they disorder that function. The arterial and venous circulations become more rapid by active exercise, and which concludes by giving greater force to the tissue of the heart. It is the same with respiration and calorification. The same takes place with regard to nutrition, a function which exercise increases, not only in the muscles in movement, as we have just seen, but also in the bones, ligaments, vessels, and nerves.

By inducing cutaneous exhalation, it promotes the expulsion of injurious agents, produces a fresh color in persons who may have become pale through a sedentary life, and, to a certain extent, renders the human constitution, by means of habit, proof against the action of surrounding objects. The local effects of excessive action, or those which take place in the members themselves, are, as before observed, inflammation of the muscles, rheumatism, like that arising from cold, and inflammation of the serous articular membranes. The general effects of excessive exercise may, in the same manner as all physical and moral stimulants, exhaust the vital faculties too quickly, communicate too much rigidity to the fibres, render the vessels varicose, bring on chronic rheumatism, destroy the freshness of the skin, blight the flower of youth, and produce old age and death before the time ordained by nature.

Ancient writers inform us that it was a rare thing to meet with athletes, who, having signalized themselves from their earliest youth in gymnastic combats, were of so excellent a constitution as to be able, when they had reached a more advanced age, to acquire the same honors in contending for the prize with grown men. Aristotle assures us, that amongst the conquerors in the Olympic Games, not more than two or three at the most could be found to whom nature had granted such an advantage.

In relation to the mental or thinking system, "every movement," says Cabanis, "becomes in its turn the principle or occasion of new impressions, of which the frequent repetition and the varied character must increase more and more the circle of our judgments, or tend unceasingly to rectify them. It hence follows that labor, giving to this word the most general signification, cannot but have an influence infinitely useful on the habits of the understanding, and consequently also on those of the will." This argument is evidently applicable to varied exercise. On the contrary, "the great division of labor, so favorable to the perfecting of the arts, contracts more and more the understanding of workmen." Exercises, moreover, inspire confidence in difficult situations, and suggests resources in danger. Their consequent influence upon the moral conduct of man is such, that, by a courage which is well founded, because it springs from a perfect knowledge of his own powers, he is often enabled to render the most important services to others.

Although the direct effect of exercise is not only to confer power on the muscular and other organs, but to multiply external impressions, and to occupy with them all the senses at once; still minds thus disposed, in general occupy themselves rather with objects of imagination and sentiment, than with those which demand more complicated operation. The sense of muscular power impresses determinations which, carrying man perpetually out of himself, scarcely permit him to dwell upon impressions transmitted to his brain. The only action of that organ, during these exercises, seems to be limited to ordering the movements.

Hence, exercise, especially taken in the open air, amidst new and varied objects of sight, is not favorable to reflection—to labors which demand the assemblage and concentration of all the powers of the mind. It is, on the contrary, in the absence of external impressions, that we become more capable of seizing many relations, and of following a long train of purely abstract reasoning. As life spent chiefly in active muscular exercises would leave in a state of repose those central organs that are subservient to the moral qualities and intellectual faculties, I agree with Seneca and Camper, in proscribing all such exercises, or such degrees of exercise, as would exhaust the mind, and render man incapable of aptitude in science, polite literature, and art.

The cultivation of bodily strength, in preference to every thing else, would establish only the right of the strongest, as it is found to exist in the origin of society. To cultivate the faculties of the mind exclusively, would produce only the weakness of sentiment or excess of passion. There is,

2*

for every individual, a means of making all these dispositions act in harmony; and the due blending of physical
and moral education alone can produce it. Let it be remembered that young persons will much more easily be
withdrawn from the application they ought to pay to the
study of the sciences, by insipid recreations and trifling
games, than by the fatiguing exercises necessary for their
development and the preservation of their health, which,
however, habit soon renders easy and delightful. To what
vices do not a sedentary life and the practice of gaming
give rise?—whilst well-regulated exercises excite ambition
to excel, and energy in the performance of every duty.

The philosophers of antiquity, such as Aristotle and
Plato, regarded gymnastic exercises as of vast importance,
and considered a state defective and badly organized where
these exercises were not instituted. Colleges, called
Gymnasia, were therefore, established everywhere, and
superintended by distinguished masters. Accordingly, the
illustrious men of the Grecian and Roman republics, even
those who shone in literature and the fine arts, received
the same physical education. The gymnastic exercises
which are here recommended are not intended to produce
athletes, but to strengthen the human constitution. One
exercise gives solidity, another address; and we may even
say that the various kinds of exercise are sometimes opposed
to each other. The strongest peasant is far from being the
best runner; and the most vigorous dancer would probably
be deficient in strength. There is, however, a mean to be
found in the disposition of every individual to preserve
both skill and strength, and this is what ought to be
sought. For this purpose, it will suffice to practise young
persons a few hours every day, sometimes at one exercise,
and sometimes at another.

GENERAL DIRECTIONS.

It only remains for us to give a few directions as to the time, place, and circumstances of exercise. The best time for the elementary exercises is when the air is cool, as, even in summer, it is early in the morning, or after the sun has declined; and they should never immediately follow a meal. The best place for these elementary exercises is a smooth grass-plat, or a firm sandy sea-beach. Chasms, stones, and stakes, are always dangerous. At the commencement, the coat and all unnecessary clothes should be laid aside; and all hard or sharp things should be taken from the pockets of the remaining dress. A very light covering on the head, as a straw hat, is best; the shirt-collar should be open, the breast being either exposed or thinly covered; the waistband of the trousers should not be tight, and the boots or shoes should have no iron about them.

As sudden transitions are always bad, exercise should begin gently, and should terminate in the same manner. The left hand and arm being commonly weaker than the right, they should be exercised till they become as strong. This custom is advantageous, not only for all military and mechanical gymnastic exercises, but also for all their operations. The being cooled too quickly is injurious. Therefore, drinking when very hot, or lying down on the cold ground, should be carefully avoided. No exertion should be carried to excess, as that only exhausts and enfeebles the body. Therefore, whenever the gymnast feels tired, or falls behind his usual mark, he should resume his clothes, and walk home. The moment exercise is finished, the clothes should always be put on, and the usual precautions adopted to prevent taking cold.

The necessary fittings-up of an exercising ground are a leaping stand, a vaulting horse, a balancing bar, a climbing stand, with ladders, poles, and ropes, which may be seen united as simply and economically as possible, in a subsequent sketch—(Plate XVIII. CLIMBING.)

In most exercises, a belt or cincture is of utility; and it seems, in all ages, to have been naturally employed. The weakest savage, who could not follow others in the course without panting, would find, by placing his hand over his abdomen, and supporting the liver and other organs which descend into that cavity, that he was aided in running, and breathed more easily; and thence he would make for himself a belt. United in societies, men would still preserve their belt, though it might not seem particularly advantageous, except to those whose active mode of life approached a primitive state, such as travellers, couriers, and porters.

The Greeks put on their belts before they commenced wrestling; and many physicians, both ancient and modern, recommend the use of belts, as being to the whole of the body, and to the parts over which they are placed, what the exterior sheaths or aponeuroses are to the muscles— bands which embrace and keep firm the parts over which they are placed. The common belt has leathern straps, and buckles to fasten it, an iron ring and a pocket. A double cincture for wrestling forms a very strong girth, which is put on by pupils who are very strong, when they wrestle. These belts may be made of different sizes, for youths of different ages: of five or six inches for tall youths and men, and of eight or ten inches for wrestlers. Their length is in proportion to the size of the person who uses them. These belts are very useful in strengthening the abdominal region in running and leaping. Riders, also, should furnish themselves with belts before getting on horseback, to prevent too violent motion of the viscera of the abdomen, and the disorders which may result from it. The use, indeed, of belts will by degrees prove their utility, and they will probably be worn even externally, without reference to physical exercises. They deserve this the more, because they give an air of lightness and elegance to the shape, and develope the chest.

The most useful thing in existence is dangerous, if improperly applied. In very young persons, the chest and abdomen have been compressed by fastening the belt too tight, or making it too wide; and disorders of digestion and respiration have consequently been caused by pushing in the false ribs. This is an imprudence that should be avoided. If the belt be too low, it may press too much on the lower part of the belly; if too high, it may disorder the chest. It must therefore be placed on the loins, so as to pass over the navel; and, as said before, it must not be too tight. Having given these ideas of the utility of belts, and the manner of using them, it remains only to explain the triple use of those adopted for exercises : 1st, they fulfill, by their size and other circumstances, all the conditions which render them useful; 2d, a pocket serves to inclose the articles that may be wanted, according to the class of exercises performing; 3d, an iron ring is intended to suspend, by means of hooks, any thing we wish to carry, so as to leave the hands at liberty.

TRAINING.

This is important in relation to various exercises to be described. The art of training for athletic exercises, or laborious exertions, consists in purifying the body and strengthening its powers, by certain processes, which are now to be described. The advantages of it, however, are not confined to pedestrians, wrestlers, or pugilists; they extend to every one: for, were training generally introduced, instead of medicine, for the prevention and cure of diseases, its beneficial consequences would assuredly prolong life, and promote its happiness. Every physiologist knows that all the parts which compose the human body—solids as well as liquids—are successively absorbed and deposited. Hence ensues a perpetual renovation of them, regulated by the nature of our food and general habits. The health of all the parts, and the soundness of their structure, depend on this perpetual absorption and renovation. Now, nothing so effectually as exercise excites at once absorption and secretion. It accordingly promotes all the vital functions without hurrying them, renovates all the parts, and preserves them apt and fit for their offices.

It follows, then, that health, vigor, and activity, chiefly depend upon exercise and regimen; or, in other words, upon the observance of those rules which constitute the theory of training. The effect has accordingly corresponded with the cause assigned in this view of the subject, in every instance where it has been adopted; and, although not commonly resorted to as the means of restoring invalids to health, there is every reason to believe that it would prove effectual in curing many obstinate diseases, such as bilious complaints, obesity, gout, and rheumatism.

The Ancients entertained this opinion. They were, says a popular writer on medicine, by no means unacquainted with or inattentive to these instruments of medicine, although modern practitioners appear to have no idea of removing disease, or restoring health, but by pouring drugs into the stomach. Heroditus is said to have been the first who applied the exercises and regimen of the Gymnasium to the removal of disease, or the maintenance of health. Among the Romans, Asclepiades carried this so far, that he is said, by Celsus, almost to have banished the use of internal remedies from his practice. He was the inventor of various modes of exercise and gestation, in Rome. In his own person, he afforded an excellent example of the wisdom of his rules, and the propriety of his regimen. Pliny tells us that, in early life, he made a public profession, that he would agree to forfeit all pretensions to the name of a physician, should he ever suffer from sickness, or die but of old age; and, what is extraordinary, he fulfilled his promise, for he lived upwards of a century, and at last was killed by a fall down stairs.

As to the locomotive system, modern experience sufficiently proves that exercise is the most powerful strengthener of the muscles, and of every part on which activity depends. In its operation on the vital system, training always appears to benefit the state of the lungs. Indeed, one of its most striking effects is to improve the wind: that is, to enable a man to draw a larger inspiration, and to hold his breath longer. As to the intellectual system, Sir J. Sinclair observes, that, by training, the mental faculties are also improved; the attention being more ready, and the perception more acute, owing probably to the clearness of the stomach, and better digestion.

It must, therefore, be admitted, that the most beneficial consequences to general health arise from training. The simplicity of the rules for it is assuredly a great recommendation to a trial of the experiment. The whole process may be resolved into the following principles:—1st, the evacuating, which cleanses the stomach and intestines;

2nd, the sweating, which takes off the superfluities of fat and humours; 3rd, the daily course of exercise, which improves the wind and strengthens the muscles; and, lastly, the regimen, which nourishes and invigorates the body. To those who are to engage in corporeal exercises beyond their ordinary powers, it is indispensably necessary. Pedestrians, therefore, who are matched either against others or against time, and pugilists who engage to fight, must undergo the training process before they contend. The issue of the contest, if their powers be nearly equal, will, in a great measure, depend upon their relative condition, as effected by training, at the hour of trial.

Training was known to the ancients, who paid much attention to the means of augmenting corporeal vigor and activity. Accordingly, among the Greeks and Romans, certain rules of exercise and regimen were prescribed to the candidates for gymnastic celebrity. We are assured, that, among the Greeks, previously to the solemn contests at the public games, the strictest temperance, sobriety, and regularity in living, were indispensably requisite. The candidates were, at the same time, subjected to daily exercise in the Gymnasium, which continued during ten months, and which, with the prescribed regimen, constituted the preparatory training adopted by the athletæ of Greece. Among the Romans, the exercises of the palæstra degenerated from the rank of a liberal art, and became a profession, which was embraced only by the lowest of mankind; the exhibitions of the gladiators being bloody and ferocious spectacles, which evinced the barbarous taste of the people. The combatants, however, were regularly trained by proper exercise, and a strict observance of regimen. Pure and salubrious air was deemed a chief requisite. Accordingly, the principal schools of their athletæ were established at Capua and Ravenna, the most healthy places in Italy; and previous to entering on this regimen, the men were subjected to the evacuating process, by means of emetics, which they preferred to purgatives.

In the more early stages of training, their diet consisted of dried figs, new cheese, and boiled grain. Afterwards animal food was introduced as a part of the athletic regimen, and pork was preferred to any other. Galen, indeed, asserts, that pork contains more real nutriment than flesh of any other kind, which is used as food by man. This fact, he' adds, is decidedly proved by the example of the athletæ, who, if they live but for one day on any other kind of food, find their vigor manifestly impaired the next. The preference given to pork by the ancients, however, does not correspond with the practice of modern trainers, who entirely reject it; but in the manner of preparing the food, they exactly agree—roasting or broiling being by both preferred to boiling, and bread unfermented to that prepared by leaven. A very small quantity of liquid was allowed to the athletæ, and this was principally water. They exercised in the open air, and became familiarized by habit to every change of the weather, the vicissitudes of which soon ceased to affect them.

To exercise their patience, and accustom them to bear pain without flinching, they were occasionally flogged on the back with the branches of a kind of rhododendron, till the blood flowed. By diminishing the quantity of the circulating liquid, this rough kind of cupping was also considered salutary ! as obviating the tendency to plethora or redundancy of blood, to which they were peculiarly liable —a proof, if true, of the nourishing qualities of their food.

When the daily exercises of the athletæ were finished, they were refreshed by immersion in a tepid bath, where

3

the perspiration and sordes—scurf, pustules, or filthy adhesions—were carefully removed from the surface of the body by the use of the strygil.* The skin was then diligently rubbed dry, and again anointed with oil. If thirsty, they were permitted to drink a small quantity of warm water. They then took their principal repast, after which they used no more exercise that day. They occasionally also went into the cold bath in the morning. They were permitted to sleep as many hours as they chose; and great increase of vigor, as well as of bulk, was supposed to be derived from long-continued and sound repose.† The sexual intercourse was strictly prohibited.

The manner of training among the ancients bears some resemblance to that practised by the moderns. Perhaps it is because their mode of living and general habits were somewhat different from those of the present age, that a difference of treatment is now required to produce the same effects. The great object of training for running or boxing matches, is to increase the muscular strength, and to improve the free action of the lungs, or wind, of the person subjected to the process. Seeing that the human body is so capable of being altered and renovated, it is not surprising that the art of training should be carried to a degree of perfection almost incredible; and that, by certain processes, the muscular power, the breath (or wind,) and the courage of man, should be so greatly improved as to enable him to perform the most severe or laborious undertakings.

That such effects have been produced is unquestionable:

* For this instrument, rough coarse clothes are adopted, but not with advantage.

† Little sleep is now prescribed; but its quantity should depend upon circumstances of fatigue, &c.

they are fully exemplified in the astonishing exploits of our most celebrated pedestrians and pugilists, which are the infallible results of such preparatory discipline. The skillful trainer attends to the state of the bowels, the lungs, and the skin ; and he uses such means as will reduce the fat, and at the same time invigorate the muscular fibre. The patient is purged by drastic medicines; he is sweated by walking under a load of clothes, and by lying between feather beds; and his limbs are roughly rubbed. His diet is beef or mutton ; his drink strong ale. He is gradually inured to exercise, by repeated trials in walking and running. By extenuating the fat, emptying the cellular substance, hardening the muscular fibre, and improving the breath, a man of the ordinary frame may be made to fight for one hour, with the utmost exertion of strength and courage, or to go over one hundred miles in twenty-four hours.

The most effectual process for training appears to be that practised by Captain Barclay, which has not only been sanctioned by professional men, but has met with the unqualified approbation of amateurs. We are here, therefore, almost entirely indebted to it for details. According to this method, the pedestrian, who may be supposed in tolerable condition, enters upon his training with a regular course of physic, which consists of three doses. Glauber's salts are generally preferred; and from one ounce and a half to two ounces are taken each time, with an interval of four days between each dose. After having gone through the course of physic, he commences his regular exercise, which is gradually increased as he proceeds in the training.

When the object in view is the accomplishment of a pedestrian match, his regular exercise may be from twenty to twenty-four miles a day. He must rise at five in the morning, run half a mile at the top of his speed up-hill, and then walk six miles at a moderate pace, coming in about seven to breakfast, which should consist of beef-steaks or mutton-chops under-done, with stale bread and old beer. After breakfast, he must again walk six miles at a moderate pace, and at twelve lie down in bed, without his clothes, for half an hour. On getting up, he must walk four miles, and return by four to dinner, which should also be beef-steaks or mutton-chops, with bread and beer, as at breakfast. Immediately after dinner, he must resume his exercise, by running half a mile at the top of his speed, and walking six miles at a moderate pace. He takes no more exercise for that day, but retires to bed about eight; and next morning he proceeds in the same manner.

Animal diet, it will be observed, is, according to this system, alone prescribed, and beef and mutton are preferred. All fat and greasy substances are prohibited, as they induce bile, and consequently injure the stomach. The lean of meat contains more nourishment than the fat ; and in every case, the most substantial food is preferable to any other kind. Fresh meat is the most wholesome and nourishing. Salt, spiceries, and all kinds of seasonings, with the exception of vinegar, are prohibited. The lean, then, of fat beef cooked in steaks, with very little salt, is the best ; and it should be rather under-done than otherwise. Mutton, being reckoned easy of digestion, may be occasionally given, to vary the diet and gratify the taste. The legs of fowls are also esteemed.

It is preferable to have the meat broiled, as much of its nutritive quality is lost by roasting or boiling. It ought to be dressed so as to remain tender and juicy ; for it is by these means that it will be easily digested, and afford most nourishment. Biscuit and stale bread are the only preparations of vegetable matter which are permitted to be given; and everything inducing flatulency must be carefully avoided. In general, the quantity of aliment is not limited by the trainer, but left entirely to the discretion of the pedestrian, whose appetite should regulate him in this respect.

With respect to liquors, they must be always taken cold; and home-brewed beer, old, but not bottled, is the best. A little red wine, however, may be given to those who are not fond of malt liquor; but never more than half a pint after dinner. It is an established rule to avoid liquids as much as possible; and no more liquor of any kind is allowed to be taken than is requisite to quench the thirst.

After having gone on in this regular course for three or four weeks, the pedestrian must take a four mile-sweat, which is produced by running four miles in flannel, at the top of his speed. Immediately on returning, a hot liquor is prescribed, in order to promote the perspiration; and of this he must drink one English pint. It is termed the sweating liquor, and is composed of one ounce of carraway seed, half an ounce of coriander seed, one ounce of root-liquorice, and half an ounce of sugar-candy, mixed with two bottles of cider, and boiled down to one-half. He is then put to bed in his flannels, and, being covered with six or eight pair of blankets, and a feather bed, must remain in this state from twenty-five to thirty minutes, when he is taken out, and rubbed perfectly dry. Being then well wrapt in his great coat, he walks out gently for two miles, and returns to breakfast, which, on such occasions, should consist of a roasted fowl. He afterwards proceeds with his usual exercise.

These sweats are continued weekly, till within a few days of the performance of the match; or, in other words, he must undergo three or four of these operations. If the stomach of the pedestrian be foul, an emetic or two must be given about a week before the conclusion of the training. He is now supposed to be in the highest condition.

Besides his usual or regular exercise, a person under training ought to employ himself, in the intervals, in every kind of exertion which tends to activity, such as golf, cricket, bowls, throwing quoits, &c., so that, during the whole day, both body and mind may be constantly occupied. Although the chief parts of the system depend upon sweating, exercise, and feeding, yet the object to be obtained by the pedestrian would be defeated, if these were not adjusted each to the other, and to his constitution. The trainer, before he proceeds to apply his theory, should make himself acquainted with the constitution and habits of his patient, that he may be able to judge how far he can, with safety, carry on the different parts of the process. The nature of the patient's disposition should also be known, that every cause of irritation may be avoided; for, as it requires great patience and perseverance to undergo training, every expedient to soothe and encourage the mind should be adopted.

The skillful trainer will, moreover, constantly study the progress of his art, by observing the effect of its processes, separately and in combination. If a man retain his health and spirits during the process, improve in wind, and increase in strength, it is certain that the object aimed at will be obtained; but, if otherwise, it is to be apprehended that some defect exists, through the unskillfulness or mismanagement of the trainer, which ought instantly to be remedied by such alterations as the circumstances of the case may demand. It is evident, therefore, that in many instances the trainer must be guided by his judgment, and that no fixed rules of management can, with absolute certainty, be depended upon, for producing an invariable and determinate result. In general, however, it may be calculated, that the known rules are adequate to the purpose, if the pedestrian strictly adhere to them, and the trainer bestow a moderate degree of attention to his state and condition during the progress of training.

It is impossible to fix any precise period for the completion of the training process, as it depends upon the previous condition of the pedestrian; but from two to three months, in most cases, will be sufficient, especially if he be in tolerable condition at the commencement, and possessed of sufficient perseverance and courage to submit cheerfully to the privations and hardships to which he must unavoidably be subjected. The criterion by which it may be known whether a man is in good condition—or, what is the same thing, whether he has been properly trained—is the state of the skin, which becomes smooth, elastic, and well-colored or transparent. The flesh is also firm; and the person trained feels himself light, and full of spirits. In the progress of the training, his condition may also be ascertained by the effect of the sweats, which cease to reduce his weight; and by the manner in which he performs one mile at the top of his speed. It is as difficult to run a mile at the top of one's speed as to walk a hundred; and therefore, if he perform this short distance well, it may be concluded that his condition is perfect, or that he has derived all the advantages which can possibly result from the training process.

A few words may be here added on the comparative strength of different races of men. In order to procure some exact results on this point, Peron took with him on his voyage, an instrument called a dynamometer, so con-

structed as to indicate on a dial-plate the relative force of
individuals submitted to experiment. He directed his
attention to the strength of the arms and of the loins,
making trial with several individuals of each of the races
among whom he then was, viz., twelve natives of Van
Diemen's Land, seventeen of New Holland, fifty-six of the
Island of Timor, seventeen Frenchmen belonging to the
expedition, and fourteen Englishmen in the colony of New
South Wales. The following numbers express the mean
result in each case, but all the details are given in a tabular
form in the original :—

		Strength of the Arms. Kilogrammes.	Strength of the Loins. Myriagrammes.
1.	Van Diemen's Land	50.6	
2.	New Holland	50.8	10.2
3.	Timor	58.7	11.6
4.	French	69.2	15.2
5.	English	71.4	16.3

The highest numbers in the first and second class were,
respectively, 60 and 62; the lowest in the English trials
63, and the highest 83, for the strength of the arms. In
the power of the loins, the highest among the New Hol-
landers was 13; the lowest of the English 12.7, and the
highest 21.3. "These results," observes Mr. Lawrence,
"offer the best answer to declamations on the degeneracy
of civilized man. The attribute of superior physical strength,
so boldly assumed by the eulogists of the savage state, has
never been questioned or doubted. Although we have
been consoled for this supposed inferiority by an enumeration of the many precious benefits derived from civilization,
it has always been felt as a somewhat degrading disadvantage. Bodily strength is a concomitant of good health,
which is produced and supported by a regular supply of
wholesome and nutritious food, and by active occupation.

The industrious and well-fed middle classes of a civilized community may, therefore, be reasonably expected to surpass, in this endowment, the miserable savages, who are never well-fed, and too frequently depressed by absolute want and all other privations."

POSITION.

Before entering into a detail of exercises, it is necessary to attend to what is termed position.—A standing position is the action by which we keep ourselves up. Indeed, this state, in which the body appears in repose, is itself an exercise, for it consists in a continued effort of many muscles; and the explanation we shall give of it will much facilitate that of walking.

Every one has observed that during sleep, or a fainting fit, the head inclines forward and falls upon the breast. In this case, it is in accordance with the laws of gravity; for the head, resting upon the vertebræ which support it at a point of its basis which is nearer the posterior than anterior part, cannot remain in an upright position in standing, except by an effort of the muscles at the back of the neck: it is the cessation of this effort that causes it to fall forward. The body also is unable to remain straight without fatigue. The vertebral column being placed behind, all the viscera or parts contained by the chest and belly are suspended in front of it, and would force it to bend forward unless strong muscular fibres held it back. A proof of this may be seen in pregnant and dropsical women, who are compelled, in consequence of the anterior part of the body being heavier than usual, to keep the vertebral column more fixed, and even thrown backward. The same observation may be made with regard to the pelvis basin, or lowest part of the trunk, which by its conformation would bend upon the thighs, if not kept back by the great mass of muscular fibres that form the hips. In front of the thighs, again, are the muscles which, by keeping the kneepan in position, are the means of preventing the leg from bending. Lastly, the muscles forming the calves, by contracting, are the means of preventing the leg from bending upon the foot.

Such is the general mechanism of the standing position. It is, therefore, as we observed, a concurrence of efforts: almost all the extending muscles are in a state of contraction all the time that this position is maintained, and the consequence is, a fatigue which cannot be endured for any great length of time. Hence we see persons in a standing position rest the weight of their body, first on one foot, then on another, for the purpose of procuring momentary ease to certain muscles. For this reason, also, standing still is more fatiguing than walking, in which the muscles are alternately contracted and extended.

A question of importance on this subject is, what position of the feet affords the greatest solidity in standing? We will not enter into detail of the numerous controversies by which some have defended or repudiated the position with the toes turned forward or outward: it will be sufficient to state the fact, that the larger the base of support, the firmer and more solid will the position be, and to adopt, as a *fundamental* one, the military position, which has been found practically the best by those who have nothing else to do but to walk. The equal squareness of the shoulders and body to the front, is the first great principle of position. The heels must be in a line, and closed; the knees straight; the toes turned out, with the feet forming an angle of sixty degrees; the arms hanging close to the body; the elbows turned in, and close to the sides; the hands open to the front, with the view of preserving the elbow in the position above described; the little fingers lightly touching the clothing of the limbs, with the thumb close to the forefinger; the belly rather drawn in, and the breast advanced, but without constraint; the body upright, but inclining forward, so that the weight of it may principally bear upon the fore part of the feet; the head erect, and the eyes straight to the front—(as in Plate I. fig. 1.)

To these brief directions I must add, that, in standing, the whole figure should be in such a position that the ear, shoulder, haunch, knee, and ankle are all in a line; that it must be stretched as much as possible, by raising the back of the head, drawing in the chin, straightening the spine, rising on the hips, and extending the legs; that the object of keeping the back thus straight is to allow of standing longer without fatigue; that it is important to expand the chest, and to throw the shoulders back, with the shoulder-blades, or scapulæ, quite flat behind; and that though, in military instructions, the body is thus inclined forward in standing without arms, yet when these are assumed, the body is immediately thrown about two inches backward, into a nearly perpendicular position. This position, therefore, will be modified in walking, and especially in ordinary walking; but it is an excellent fundamental position, and it cannot be too accurately acquired.

This is the amount of the drill-sergeant's instructions as to position, though this last part is omitted in the Manual describing the Field Exercise and Evolutions of the Army.

EXTENSION MOTIONS.

In order to supple the figure, open the chest, and give freedom to the muscles, the first three movements of the extension motions, as laid down for the sword exercise, are ordered to be practised. It is indeed, observed, that too many methods cannot be used to improve the carriage, and banish a rustic air; but that the greatest care must be taken not to throw the body backward instead of forward, as being contrary to every true principle of movement. I accordingly here introduce these extension motions, adding the fourth and fifth, and prefixing to each the respective word of command, in order that they may be the more distinctly and accurately executed.

Attention.—The body is to be erect, the heels close together, and the hands hanging down on each side. First Extension motion.—This serves as a caution, and the motions tend to expand the chest, raise the head, throw back the shoulders, and strengthen the muscles of the back.

One—Bring the hands and arms to the front, the fingers lightly touching at the points, and the nails downwards; then raise them in a circular direction well above the head, the ends of the fingers still touching, the thumbs pointing to the rear, the elbows pressed back, and shoulders kept down. (Plate I. fig. 2.)

Two—Separate and extend the arms and fingers, forcing them obliquely back, till they come .extended on a line with the shoulders; and as they fall gradually from thence to the original position of Attention, endeavor, as much as possible, to elevate the neck and chest. These two motions should be frequently practised, with the head turned as much as possible to the right or left, and the body kept

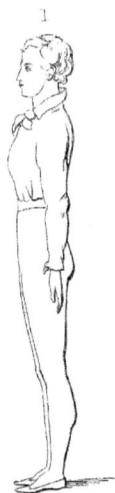

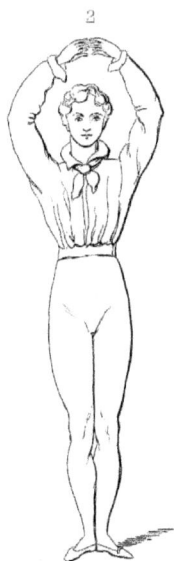

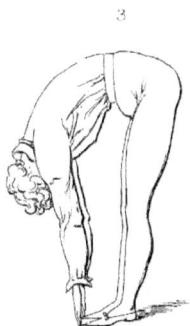

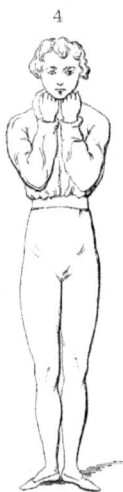

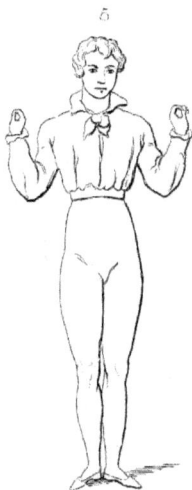

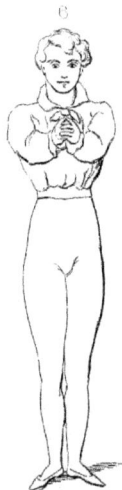

square to the front: this tends very materially to supple the neck, &c.

Three—Turn the palms of the hands to the front, pressing back the thumbs with the arms extended, and raise them to the rear, till they meet above the head; the fingers pointing upwards, with the ends of the thumbs touching.

Four—Keep the arms and knees straight, and bend over from the hips till the hands touch the feet, the head being brought down in the same direction. (Plate I. fig. 3.)

Five—With the arms flexible and easy from the shoulders, raise the body gradually, so as to resume the position of Attention. The whole should be done very gradually, so as to feel the exertion of the muscles throughout. To these extension motions, drill-sergeants, in their instructions, add the following:

One—the forearms are bent upon the arms upward and toward the body, having the elbows depressed, the shut hands touching on the little-finger sides, and the knuckles upward, the latter being raised as high as the chin, and at the distance of about a foot before it. (Plate I. fig. 4.)

Two—While the arms are thrown forcibly backward, the forearms are as much as possible bent upon the arms, and the palmar sides of the wrists are turned forward and outward (Plate I. fig. 5.) The two motions are to be repeatedly and rather quickly performed. A modification of the same movement is performed as a separate extension motion, but may be given in continuation, with the numbers following these, as words of command.

Three—The arms are extended at full length in front, on a level with the shoulder, the palms of the hands in contact. (Plate I. fig. 6.)

Four—Thus extended, and the palms retaining their

4

vertical position, the arms are thrown forcibly backward, so that the backs of the hands may approach each other as nearly as possible. These motions, also, are to be repeatedly and rather quickly performed. Another extension motion, similarly added, consists in swinging the right arm in a circle, in which, beginning from the pendant position, the arm is carried upward in front, by the side of the head, and downward behind, the object being in the latter part of this course to throw it as directly backward as possible. The same is then done with the left arm. Lastly, both arms are thus exercised together. These motions are performed quickly.

THE INDIAN CLUB EXERCISE.

THE PORTION ADOPTED IN THE ARMY.

1st. A club is held by the handle, pendent on each side (Plate II. fig. 1;)—that in the right hand is carrried over the head and left shoulder, until it hangs perpendicularly on the right side of the spine (Plate II. fig. 2;) that in the left hand is carried over the former, in exactly the opposite direction (Plate II. fig. 2,) until it hangs on the opposite side; holding both clubs still pendent, the hands are raised somewhat higher than the head (Plate II. fig. 3;) with the clubs in the same position, both arms are extended outward and backward (Plate II. fig. 6;) they are lastly dropped into the first position. All this is done slowly.

2nd. Commencing from the same position, the ends of both clubs are swung upward until they are held, vertically

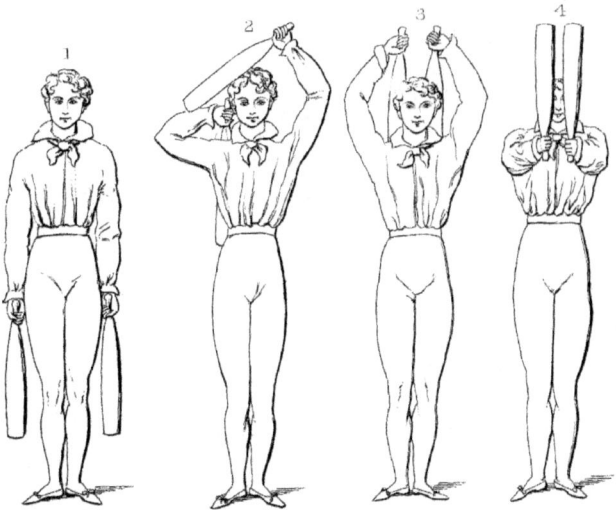

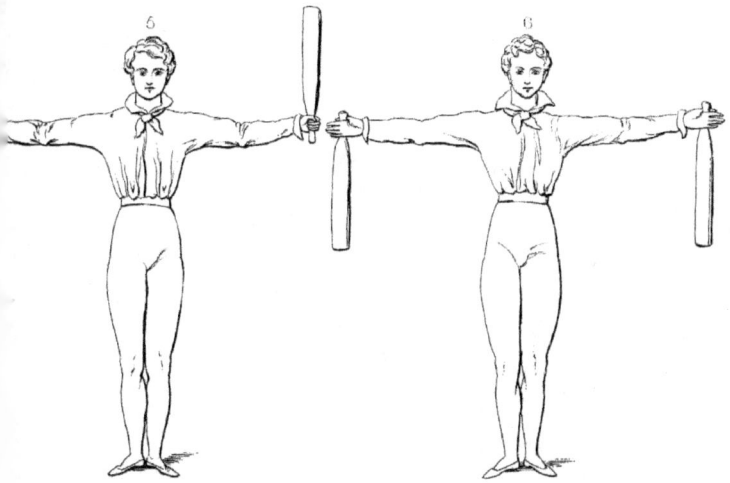

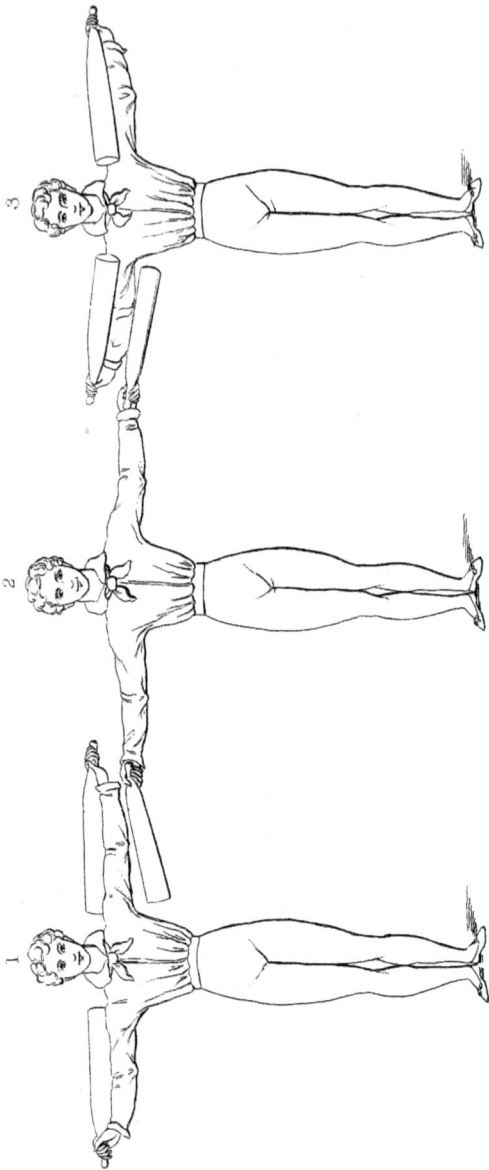

and side by side, at arm's length in front of the body, the hands being as high as the shoulders (Plate II. fig. 4;) they are next carried in the same position, at arm's length, and on the same level, as far backward as possible (Plate II. fig. 5;) each is then dropped backward until it hangs vertically downward (Plate II. fig. 6;) and this exercise ends as the first. Previous, however, to dropping the clubs backward, it greatly improves this exercise, by a turn of the wrist upward and backward, to carry the clubs into a horizontal position behind the shoulders, so that, if long enough, their ends would touch (Plate III. fig. 1;) next, by a turn of the wrist outward and downward, to carry them horizontally outward (Plate III. fig. 2;) then by a turn of the wrist upward and forward, to carry them into a horizontal position before the breast (Plate III. fig. 3;) again to carry them horizontally outward; and finally to drop them backward as already explained; and thence to the first position. All this is also done slowly.

3rd. The clubs are to be swung by the sides, first separately, and then together, exactly as the hands were in the last extension motion.

THE NEW AND MORE BEAUTIFUL PORTION NOW ADDED
FROM THE INDIAN PRACTICE.

1st. A club is held forward and upright in each hand, the fore-arm being placed horizontally, by the haunch on each side (Plate IV. fig. 1;) both are thrown in a circle upward, forward, and, by a turn of the wrist, downward and backward, so as to strike under the arms (Plate IV. fig. 2;) by an opposite movement, both are thrown back again in a similar circle, till they swing over the shoulders (Plate IV. fig. 3;) and this movement is continued as long as agreeable.

2nd. The clubs are held obliquely upward in each hand, lying on the front of the arms (Plate IV. fig. 4;) that in the right hand is allowed to fall backward (Plate IV. fig. 5,) and swings downward, forward to the extent of the arm, and as high as the head (Plate IV. fig. 6;) the moment this club begins to return from this point, in precisely the same direction, to the front of the arm, that in the left hand is allowed to drop backward, and to perform the advancing portion of this course in the time that the other performs the returning portion, so that each is at the same time swinging in an opposite direction.

3rd. From either of the first positions now given, the clubs are, by a turn of the body and extension of the arms, thrown upwards and laterally (Plate V. fig. 1;)—make, at the extent of the arms, and in front of the figure, a circle in which they sweep downward by the feet and upward over the head (Plate V. fig. 2,) and fall in a more limited curve towards the side on which they began (Plate V. fig. 3,) in such a manner that the outer one forming a circle around the shoulder and the inner one round the head, (both passing swiftly through the position in the last figure of the first exercise,) they return to the first position;—this is repeated to the other side;—and so on alternately.

4th. Beginning from either first position, the body being turned laterally,—for example, to the left, the club in the right hand is thrown upward in that direction at the full extent of the arm (Plate VI. fig. 1,) and makes the large circle in front and curve behind as in the last exercise (Plate VI. fig. 2,) while the club in the left hand makes at the same time a smaller circle in front of the head and behind the shoulders (Plate VI. figs. 1, 2, and 3,) until crossing each other before the head (rather on the right side,) their movements are exactly reversed, the club in the right hand performing the small circle round the

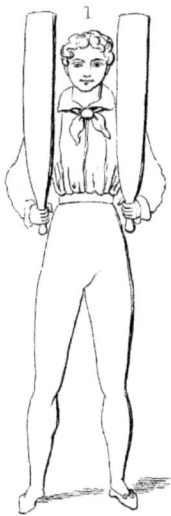

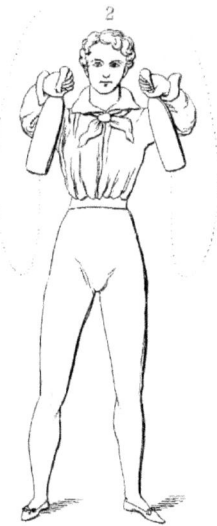

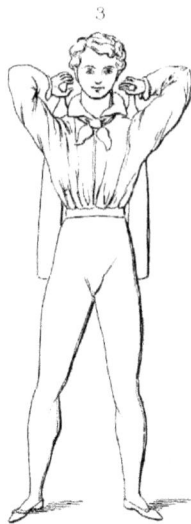

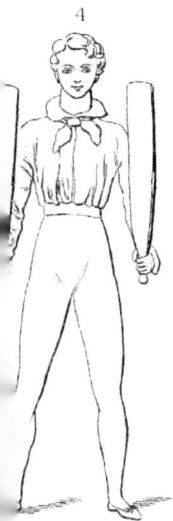

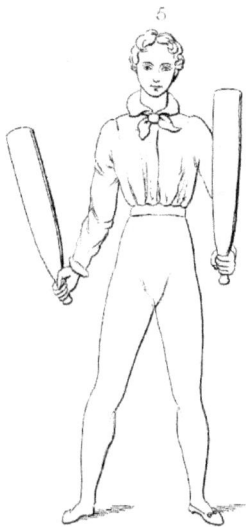

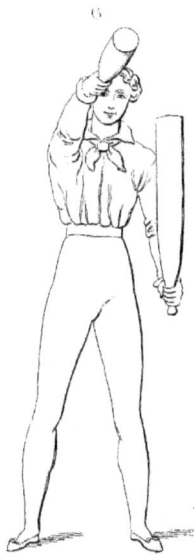

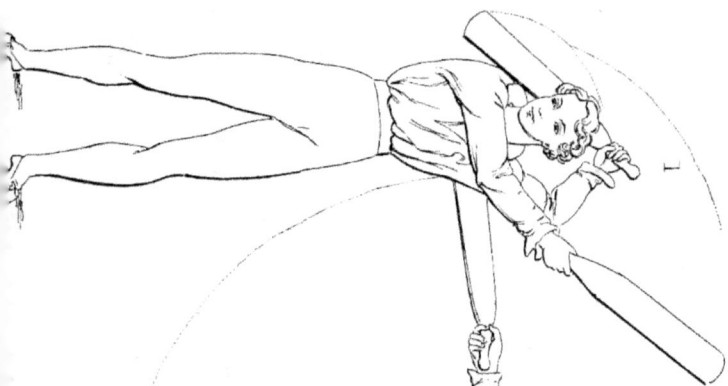

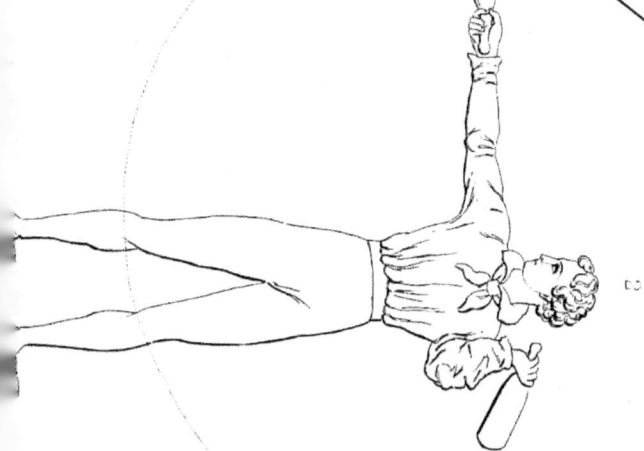

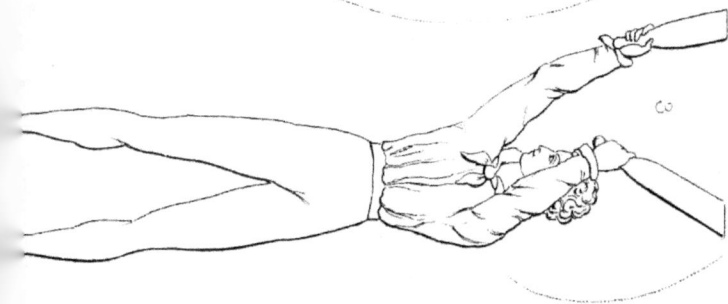

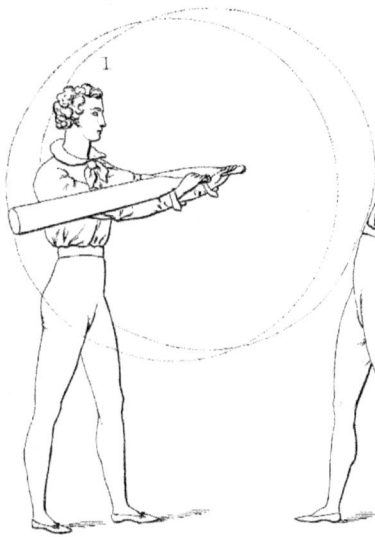

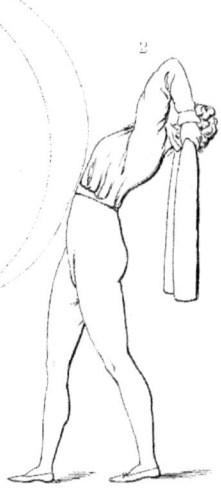

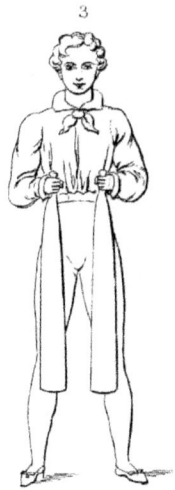

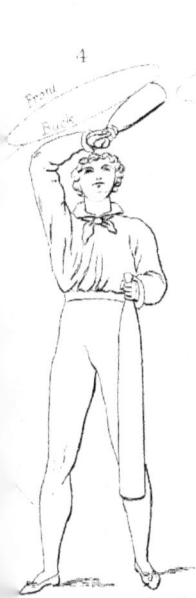

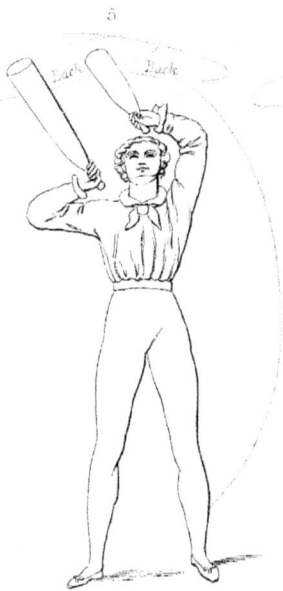

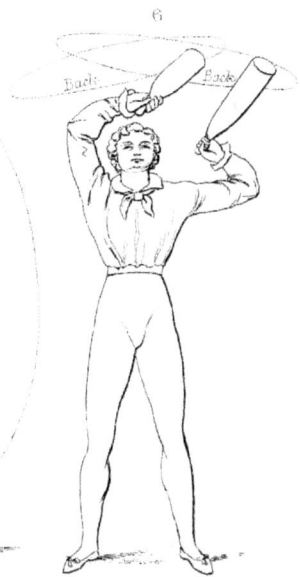

head, while that in the left performs the large one,—and these continue to be repeated to each side alternately.

5th. The clubs being in either first position, the body is turned to one side—the left for example, and the clubs being thrown out in the same direction, make each, by a turn of the wrist, a circle three times on the outer side of the outstretched arms (Plate VII. fig. 1:)—when completing the third circle, the clubs are thrown higher to the same side, sweeping together in the large circle in front, as in the second exercise, the body similarly turning to the right; but, instead of forming the smaller curve behind, both are thrown over the back (Plate VII. fig. 2;)—from this position the clubs are thrown in front, which is now toward the opposite side, and the same movements are reversed;—and so it proceeds alternately to each side.

6th. In this exercise, the clubs are reversed, both being pendent in front, but the ends of their handles being upward on the thumb sides of the hands. (Plate VII. fig. 3.) The exercise consists chiefly in describing with the ends of the clubs two circles placed obliquely to each other over the head. For this purpose, the club in the right hand is, in a sweep to that side, first elevated behind the head, and thence passing to the left (Plate VII. fig. 4,) the front, the right (Plate VII. fig. 5) behind, (where its continuation is indicated in fig. 5, and completed in fig. 6,) thus forms its circle;—meanwhile the club in the left hand, commencing when that in the right was behind the head, has passed on the back of its circle to the right, (Plate VII. fig. 5,) while that in the right hand has passed on the front of its circle to the same side (Plate VII. fig. 5, the parts performed in both being marked by complete lines, and the parts to be done merely indicated;)—and they continue, that in the right hand by the back, and that in the left hand by the front, toward the left side (Plate VII. fig. 6,) and so on at pleasure, circling over the head.

[Although but two-thirds of the body, viz., from the loins upward, are called into operation in this exercise, its importance must be estimated by the fact that they are precisely those requiring constant artificial practice, being naturally most exempted from exertion. As an adjunct to TRAINING, there is nothing in the whole round of gymnastic performances that will be found of more essential service than this exercise with the Indian clubs. It demands but little muscular exertion, and such as it does require calls chiefly upon that portion of the system which it finds in a state of comparative repose.]

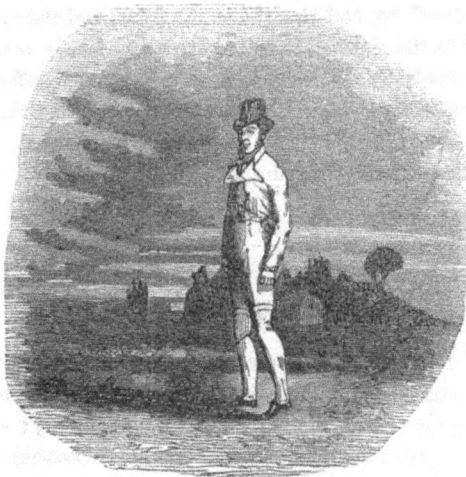

LOCOMOTIVE EXERCISES.

In Walking, the position is nearly the same as that already described under the head POSITION.

The head should be upright, easy, and capable of free motion, right, left, up, or down, without affecting the body. The body must be kept erect and square to the front, having the breast projected, and the stomach retracted, though not so as to injure either freedom of respiration or ease of attitude. The shoulders should be kept moderately and equally back and low; and the arms should hang unconstrainedly by the sides. The balance on the limbs must be perfect. The knees straight, and the toes turned out as described, the weight of the body should be thrown forward, as this facilitates progression. The military position in walking does not essentially differ from this, except in points that exclusively regard the soldier; as that the head be kept well up, and straight to the frónt, and the eyes not turned to the right or left; the arms and hands kept perfectly steady by the side, and on no account suffered to move or vibrate : care, however, being taken that the hand does not cling to the thigh, or partake in the least degree of the movement of the limb.

THE BALANCE STEP.

The object of this is to teach the free movement of the limbs, preserving at the same time perfect squareness of the shoulders, with the utmost steadiness of body; and no labor is spared to attain this first and most essential object, which forms, indeed, the very foundation of good walking. The instructor must be careful that a habit be not contracted of drooping or throwing back a shoulder at these motions, which are intended practically to show the true principles of walking, and that steadiness of body is compatible with perfect freedom in the limbs.

I.—WITHOUT GAINING GROUND.

To insure precision, the military words of command are prefixed.

Caution—Balance step without gaining ground, commencing with the left foot. The left foot is brought gently forward with the toe at the proper angle to the left, the foot about three inches from the ground, the left heel in line with the toe of the right foot.

Rear—When steady, the left foot is brought gently back (without a jerk,) the left knee a little bent, the left toe brought close to the right heel. The left foot in this posi-

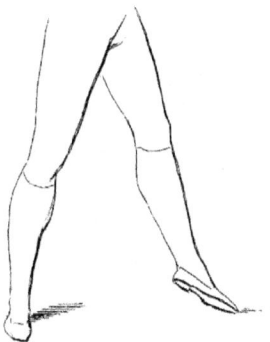

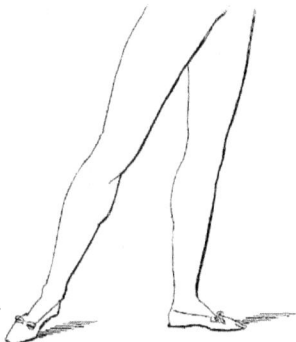

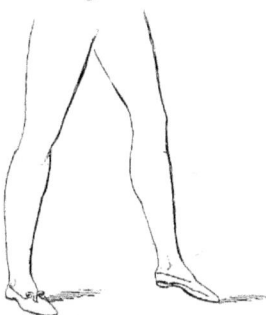

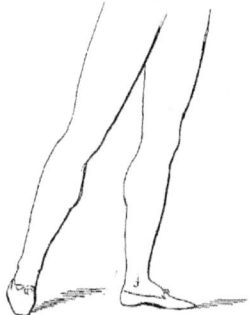

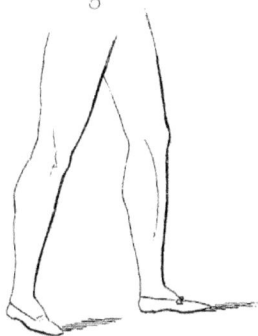

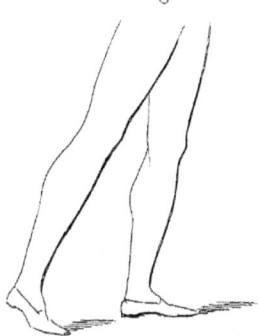

tion will not be so flat as to the front, as the toe will be a little depressed.

Front—When steady, the word Front will be given as above, and repeated to the Rear three or four times.

Halt—To prevent fatigue, the word Halt will be given, when the left foot, either advanced, or to the rear, will be brought to the right. The instructor will afterwards cause the balance to be made on the left foot, advancing and retiring the right in the same manner.

2.—GAINING GROUND BY THE WORD "FORWARD."

Front—On the word Front, the left foot is brought gently to the front, without a jerk; the knee gradually straightened as the foot is brought forward, the toe turned out a little to the left, and remaining about three inches from the ground. This posture is continued for a few seconds only in the first instance, till practice gives steadiness in the position.

Forward—On this word of command, the left foot is brought to the ground, at about thirty inches from heel to heel, while the right foot is raised at the same moment, and continues extended to the rear. The body remains upright, but inclining forward; the head erect, and neither turned to the right nor left.

Front—On the word Front, the right foot is brought forward, and so on.

WALKING.

OF all exercises, this is the most simple and easy. The weight of the body rests on one foot, while the other is advanced; it is then thrown upon the advanced foot, while the other is brought forward; and so on in succession. In this mode of progression, the slowness and equal distribution of motion is such, that many muscles are employed in a greater or less degree; each acts in unison with the rest; and the whole remains compact and united. Hence, the time of its movements may be quicker or slower, without deranging the union of the parts, or the equilibrium of the whole. It is owing to these circumstances, that walking displays so much of the character of the walker,—that it is light and gay in women and children, steady and grave in men and elderly persons, irregular in the nervous and irritable, measured in the affected and formal, brisk in the sanguine, heavy in the phlegmatic, and proud or humble, bold or timid, &c., in strict correspondence with individual character.

The utility of walking exceeds that of all other modes of progression. While the able pedestrian is independent of stage coaches and hired horses, he alone fully enjoys the scenes through which he passes, and is free to dispose of his time as he pleases. To counterbalance these advantages, greater fatigue is doubtless attendant on walking: but this fatigue is really the result of previous inactivity; for daily exercise, gradually increased, by rendering walking more easy and agreeable, and inducing its more frequent practice, diminishes fatigue in such a degree, that very great distances may be accomplished with pleasure, instead of painful exertion.

Moderate walking exercises the most agreeable influence over all the functions. In relation to health, walking accelerates respiration and circulation, increases the temperature and cutaneous exhalation, and excites appetite and healthful nutrition. Hence, as an anonymous writer observes, the true pedestrian, after a walk of twenty miles, comes in to breakfast with freshness on his countenance, healthy blood coursing in every vein, and vigor in every limb, while the indolent and inactive man, having painfully crept over a mile or two, returns to a dinner which he cannot digest. In all individuals, walking is indispensably joined with the exercise of one or more of the external senses. It receives from the cerebral faculties a powerful influence, by which it is either accelerated or prolonged. Walking upon soft even ground, at a moderate pace, is an exercise that may be taken without inconvenience, and even with advantage, after a meal. It is adapted for convalescents, who are not yet allowed to take stronger exercise. A firm, yet easy and graceful walk, is by no means common. There are few men who walk well if they have not learnt to regulate their motions by the lessons of a master, and this instruction is still more necessary for ladies. Having, now, therefore, taken a general view of the character and utility of walking, I subjoin some more particular remarks on the

GENERAL MECHANISM OF WALKING.

For the purpose of walking, we first bear upon one leg the weight of the body, which pressed equally on both. The other leg is then raised, and the foot quits the ground by rising from the heel to the point. For that purpose, the leg must be bent upon the thigh, and the thigh upon the pelvis: the foot is then carried straight forward, at a sufficient height to clear the ground without grazing it. To render it possible, however, to move this foot, the haunch, which rested with its weight upon the thigh, must turn forward and out. As soon as, by this movement, this foot has passed the other, it must be extended on the leg, and the leg upon the thigh, and in this manner, by the lengthening of the whole member, and without being drawn back, it reaches the ground at a distance in advance of the other foot, which is more considerable according to the length of the step, and it is placed so softly on the ground as not to jerk or shake the body in the slighest degree. As soon as the foot which has been placed on the ground becomes firm, the weight of the body is transported to the limb on that side, and the other foot, by a similar mechanism, is brought forward in its turn. In all walking, the most important circumstance is, that the body incline forward, and that the movement of the leg and thigh spring from the haunch, and be free and natural. Viewed in this way, the feet have been well compared to the spokes of a wheel : the weight of the body falling upon them alternately.

This exercise puts in action the extensors and flexors of the thighs and legs, a great number of the muscles of the trunk, and more or less those of the shoulders, according to the rapidity of the pace, and the greater or less degree of projection communicated to the arm, which, in this exercise, acts as a balancer of the body, the motion being exactly the reverse of that of the corresponding leg. It draws the fluids more into the inferior than superior members : it gives but little strength to the latter. Walking may be performed in three different times,—slow, moderate, or quick—which somewhat modify its action.

THE SLOW WALK, OR MARCH.

In the march, the weight of the body is advanced from the heel to the instep, and the toes are turned out. This being done, one foot, the left for instance, is advanced, with the knee straight, and the toe inclined to the ground, which, without being drawn back, it touches before the heel, in such a manner, however, that the sole, at the conclusion of the step, is nearly parallel with the ground, which it next touches with its outer edge; the right foot is then immediately raised from the inner edge of the toe, and similarly advanced, inclined, and brought to the ground; and so in succession. (Plate VIII. figs. 1 and 2.) Thus, in the march, the toe externally first touches, and internally last leaves the ground; and so marked is this tendency, that, in the stage step, which is meant to be especially dignified,—as the posterior foot acquires an awkward flexure when the weight has been thrown on the anterior,—in order to correct this, the former is for an instant extended, its toe even turned backwards and outwards, and its tip internally alone rested on the ground, previous to its being in its turn advanced. Thus the toe's first touching and last leaving the ground, is peculiarly marked in this grandest form of the march. This pace should be practised until it can be firmly and gracefully performed.

THE MODERATE AND THE QUICK PACE.

These will be best understood by a reference to the pace which we have just described; the principal difference between them being as to the advance of the weight of the body, the turning out of the toes, and the part of the foot which first touches and last leaves the ground. We shall find that the times of these two paces require a further advance of the weight, and suffer successively less and less of turning out the toes, and of this extended touching with the toe, and covering the ground with the foot.

THE MODERATE PACE.

Here the weight of the body is advanced from the heel to the ball of the foot; the toes are less turned out; and

5

it is no longer the toe, but the ball of the foot, which first
touches and last leaves the ground; its outer edge, or the
ball of the little toe, first breaking the descent of the foot,
and its inner edge, or the ball of the great toe, last projecting the weight—(Plate VIII. figs. 3 and 4.) Thus, in
this step, less of the foot may be said actively to cover
the ground; and this adoption of nearer and stronger points
of support and action is essential to the increased quickness
and exertion of the pace.

The mechanism of this pace has not been sufficiently attended to. People pass from the march to the quick pace
they know not how; and hence all the awkwardness and
embarrassment of their walk when their pace becomes moderate, and the misery they endure when this pace has to
be performed by them, unaccompanied, up the middle of a
long and well-lighted room, where the eyes of a brilliant
assembly are exclusively directed to them. Let those who
have felt this but attend to what we have here said: the
motion of the arms and of every other part depends on it.

THE QUICK PACE.

Here, the weight of the body is advanced from the heel
to the toes; the toes are least turned out; and still nearer
and stronger points of support and action are chosen. The
outer edge of the heel first touches the ground, and the sole
of the foot projects the weight.

These are essential to the increased quickness of this
pace—(Plate VIII. figs. 5 and 6;) and it is important to
remark, as to all these paces, that the weight is successively
more thrown forward, and the toes are successively less
turned out. In the grandest form of the march, the toes,
as we have seen, are, in the posterior foot, though but for
a moment, even thrown backwards; in the moderate pace,
they have an intermediate direction; and in the quick pace,

they are thrown more directly forward, as in the six figures of Plate VIII.

It is this direction of the toes, and still more the nearer and stronger points of support and action, namely, the heel and sole of the foot, which are essential to the quick pace so universally practised, but which, together with the great inclination of the body, being ridiculously transferred to the moderate pace, make unfortunate people look so awkward, as we shall now explain. The time of the moderate pace is, as it were, filled up by the more complicated process of the step—by the gradual and easy breaking of the descent of the foot on its outer edge, or the ball of the little toe, by the deliberate positing of the foot, by its equally gradual and easy projection from its inner edge, or the ball of the great toe. The quick pace, if its time be lengthened, has no such filling up: the man stumps at once down on his heel, and could rise instantly from his sole, but finds that, to fill up his time, he must pause an instant; he feels he should do something, and does not know what; his hands suffer the same momentary paralysis as his feet; he gradually becomes confused and embarrassed: deeply sensible of this, he at last exhibits it externally; a smile or a titter arises, though people do not well know at what; but, in short, the man has walked like a clown, because the mechanism of his step has not filled up its time, or answered its purpose.

I trust that the mechanism and time of the three paces are here simply, clearly, and impressively described. The following is the more imperfect, but still useful, military description, with its words of command:—

SLOW STEP.

March.—On the word March, the left foot is carried

thirty inches to the front, and, without being drawn back, is placed softly on the ground, so as not to jerk or shake the body; seventy-five of these steps to be taken in a minute. (The recruit is ordered to be carefully trained, and thoroughly instructed in this step, as an essential foundation for arriving at accuracy in the paces of more celerity. This is the slowest step at which troops are to move.)

QUICK STEP.

The cadence of the slow pace having become perfectly habitual, a quick time is next taught, which is 108 steps in a minute, each of thirty inches, making 270 feet in a minute.

Quick March.—The command Quick March being given with a pause between them, the word Quick is to be considered as a caution, and the whole to remain perfectly steady. On the word March, the whole move off, conforming to the directions already given. (This pace is applied generally to all movements by large as well as small bodies of troops; and therefore the recruit is trained and thoroughly instructed in this essential part of his duty.)

DOUBLE MARCH.

The directions for the march apply, in a great degree, to this step, which is 150 steps in a minute, each of thirty-six inches, making 450 feet in a minute.

Double March.—On the word Double March, the whole step off together with the left feet, keeping the head erect, and the shoulders square to the front; the knees are a little bent; the body is more advanced than in the other marches; the arms hang with ease down the outside of the thighs. The person marching is carefully habituated to the full pace of thirty-six inches, otherwise he gets into the habit of a short trot, which defeats the obvious advantages of this degree of march. In the army, great advantage attends the constant use of the plummet; and the several lengths swinging the times of the different marches in a minute, are as follows:—

					In Hun.
Slow time	. .	75 steps in the minute	. .	24,96
Quick time	. .	108	"	"	. .	12,03
Double March	.	150	"	"	. .	6,26

A musket ball, suspended by a string which if not subject to stretch, and on which are marked the different required lengths, answers the above purpose, may be easily acquired, and is directed to be frequently compared with an accurate standard in the adjutant's possession. The length of the plummet is to be measured from the point of suspension to the centre of the ball. In practising all these paces, the pupils should also be accustomed to march upon a narrow plane, where there is room for only one foot, upon rough uneven ground, and on soft ground which yields to the foot.

Walking exercises a greater influence over the economy when it takes place on inclined planes than on a flat surface. In ascending, the effort is made in a direction directly opposed to the general tendency of heavy bodies : the body is strongly bent, the upper part of the trunk in advance ; the action of the posterior and anterior muscles of the thigh is considerable ; and circulation and respiration are speedily accelerated by the violence of the muscular contractions. In descending, on the contrary, effort is requisite to keep up the body, which tends to obey the laws of gravitation ; and to moderate the tendency of gravity to project forward in the centre, the body is thrown back, the sacrospinal mass, and the posterior muscles of the neck, are strongly contracted, the knees bent, and the steps much shorter. Men with long flat feet, and the heel bone little projecting, are bad walkers.

FEATS IN WALKING.

The power of walking great distances without fatigue is an important matter, in which the English have of late excelled. A good walker will do six miles an hour, for one hour, on a good road.* If in perfect training, he may even do twelve miles in two hours. Eighteen miles in three hours is a much more doubtful affair, though some are said to have achieved it.

A Cork paper, of recent date, describes a match of ten miles in 120 minutes, on the Mallow and Fermoy Road, by Captain John T. G. Campbell, of the 91st (Argyleshire) Regiment, accoutred in heavy marching order of a private soldier, viz., with knapsack and kit, great-coat and mess-tin, musket, bayonet, and sixty rounds of ball cartridge : total, fifty pounds' weight. Heavy bets were pending on the issue. The captain started at eight o'clock, A. M., and performed this undertaking in the short time of 107 minutes and a quarter, thus winning the match, and having twelve minutes and three quarters to spare.

At the rate of five miles an hour, pedestrians of the first class will do forty miles in eight hours, and perhaps fifty in ten.† At the rate of four miles an hour, a man may

* Seven miles in one hour are said to have been done by some.

† A clever writer in Blackwood's Magazine says, "There can be no doubt that, out of the British army, on a war establishment, ten thousand men might be chosen, by trial, who would compose a corps capable of marching fifty miles a day, on actual service, for a whole week. The power of such a corps is not to be calculated : it would far outgo cavalry."

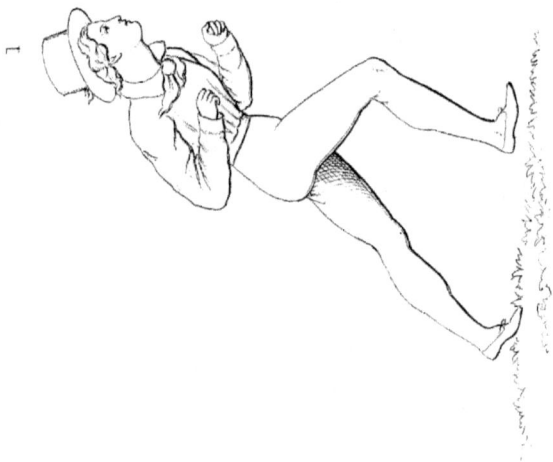

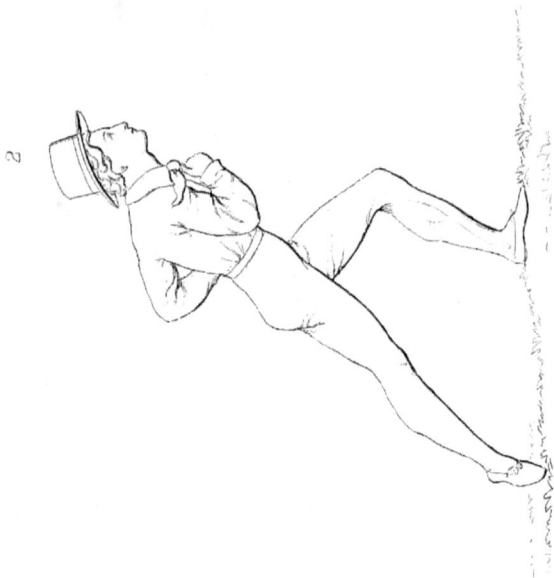

walk any length of time. Robert Skipper walked 1000 miles in 1000 successive half-hours, on the same ground Captain Barclay walked 1000 miles in 1000 successive hours.

In the art of walking quickly, the circumstance perhaps most important is, to keep the knees somewhat bent and springy.

RUNNING.

"Running," says one of our gymnasiarchs, "only differs from walking by the rapidity of the movement." This is quite incorrect. Running is precisely intermediate to walking and leaping; and, in order to pass into it from walking, the motion must be changed. A series of leaps from each foot alternately must be performed, in order to constitute it; the foot which is left behind quits the ground before the foot in advance is firmly fixed, so that the centre of gravity remains uncertain in passing from one leg to the other, which forms a series of leaps, and renders a fall a common occurrence.

POSITION IN RUNNING.

The upper part of the body is slightly inclined forward; the head slightly thrown backward, to counteract the gravity forward: the breast is freely projected; the shoulders are steady, to give a fixed point to the auxiliary muscles of respiration: the upper parts of the arm are kept near the sides; the elbows are bent, and each forms an acute angle; the hands are shut, with the nails turned inwards; and the whole arms move but slightly, in order that the muscles of respiration on the chest may be as little as possible disturbed, and follow only the impulse communicated by other parts—(Plate IX. fig. 1.) There exists, in fact, during the whole time of running, a strong and permanent contraction of the muscles of the shoulder and arm, which, though very violent, is less serviceable to the extended movements, than to keep the chest immoveable, toward which the arms are brought close, the flexors and adductors of which are especially contracted.

ACTION IN RUNNING.

At every step, the knees are stretched out; the legs kept as straight as possible; the feet almost graze the ground ; the tread is neither with the mere balls of the toes, nor with the whole sole of the foot; and the spring is made rapidly from one foot to the other, so that they pass each other with great velocity—(Plate IX. fig. 2.)

But the abdominal members are not the only ones in motion, although it is in them that the greatest development takes place. Throughout the whole time of running, a strong and permanent contraction of the muscles of the shoulder, arm, and forearm takes place; this, though very violent, is less for the purpose of aiding motion than of preserving the immobility of the thorax, which is pressed upon the whole thoracic member, whose flexors and adductors are strongly contracted. The degree of velocity, however, must be proportioned to the length of the steps. Too slow and long, as well as too quick and short, steps, may be equally injurious.

RESPIRATION.

Speed, and still more duration in running, are in proportion to the development of the lungs, and consequently the volume of oxygen and blood which they can combine in their parenchyma at each respiratory movement. Thus, of two men, one having the abdominal members developed, and the other possessing good lungs, the former will run with the greatest speed for a short distance, but if the distance be considerable, he will soon be gained upon by the latter. A runner, after performing a certain space, is seized with a difficulty of breathing, long before the repetition of the contractions has produced fatigue in the abdominal members. To excel, therefore, in running, requires, like walking and dancing, a peculiar exercise. As the muscular contractions depend, for their principle of excitement, on the respiration, the chest should be firmly fixed, so as both to facilitate this, and to serve as a point of support for the efforts of the lower members. The best runners are those who have the *best wind*, and keep the breast dilated for the longest time.

During the whole time of running, long inspirations and slow expirations are of the greatest importance; and young persons cannot be too early accustomed to them. To facilitate respiration towards the end of the race, the upper part of the body may be leant a little forward. Running should cease as soon as the breath becomes very short, and a strong perspiration takes place.

MODERATE RUNNING.

This is performed gently and in equal time, and may be extended to a considerable space. In practising this pace, it is necessary to fix the distance to be run; and this should always be proportioned to the age and strength of the runners. This exercise, more than all others, requires to be proceeded with in a progressive manner. If, at the first trial, you run too fast or too long a time, it may produce spitting of blood and headache, or aneurisms of the heart and principal vessels, especially if the weather be dry and cold.

A moderately cool day may accordingly be chosen, a distance of three hundred feet measured, and the runners placed in a line at one end. They may then start, trot at the rate of about seven feet in a second to the opposite end, turn, and continue until they reach the spot whence they started. Frequent repetition of this is sufficient at first. Afterwards, they may run over this space, two, three, or four times without stopping; and the exercise may then be limited to this. It may, on subsequent days, be extended to five, six, and seven times the distance.

Fatigue is then generally quite removed; and the run may either be continued farther, or the runners, if neither heated nor winded, may accelerate their pace. They may next attempt a mile in ten minutes; and repeat this, till, being gradually less and less heated, they can either extend the distance, or diminish the time, in any measured proportion. At this pace, six miles may afterwards be run in an hour.

RAPID RUNNING.

This is best applied to a short space in a little time. Three hundred feet upon an open plain will not generally be found too great. At each end of this, a cross line may be drawn, and the runners may arrange themselves on one line, while the umpire is placed at the other. On the latter giving the signal, the running commences, and he who first passes him gains the race. It is extremely useful always to run beyond the line at a gentler pace, as it gradually lowers the actions of the respiratory and circulating systems.

Running is more easy on a level surface, but should be

practised on ground of every variety: upon long, square, and circular plots of ground. The pupils should be accustomed to turn promptly out of the direct line—a faculty not possessed by animals, and exceedingly useful when pursued. They should also run up hill, and particularly down, as it is dangerous unless frequently practised.

FEATS IN RUNNING.

The practice of running may be carried to a great degree of perfection.

A quarter of a mile in a minute is good running; and a mile in four minutes, at four starts, is excellent.

The mile was perhaps never run in four minutes, but it has been done in four minutes and a half.*

A mile in five minutes is good running. Two miles in ten minutes is oftener failed in than accomplished. Four miles in twenty is said to puzzle the cleverest.

Ten miles an hour is done by all the best runners. Fifteen miles in an hour and a half has never perhaps been done.

It is reported that West ran forty miles in five hours and a half. This, it is said, was done by one individual in four hours and three quarters, or less.

As to great distances, Rainer failed in two attempts to accomplish 100 miles in eighteen hours. West is said to have accomplished this.

EFFECTS OF RUNNING.

In running, the mass of our organs is agitated by violent and constant shocks, which succeed with rapidity; but the abdominal members are not the only ones in motion,

---

* Half a mile was recently run in two minutes; but it was down a fall as precipitous as a mountain's side, and the performer was blind in the last twenty yards.—ED. Fifth Edition.

although they are those in which the development is most considerable. Running developes not only the abdominal members, but has a strong influence upon the respiratory parts. This exercise is particularly suited to young persons, especially those of a lymphatic temperament. It should not, however, be practised after meals.

LEAPING.

Leaping consists principally in the sudden straightening of the articulations, performed by a strong and instantaneous contraction of the extensors, by which the body is rapidly projected from the ground.

The leaping-stand consists of two moveable posts, above six feet high, having, above the second foot from the ground, holes bored through them, at the distance of an inch from each other; two iron pins to be placed in the holes at any height; a cord, at least ten feet long, passed over these pins, and kept straight by two sand-bags at its ends; and weights upon the feet of the posts, to prevent them from falling—(Plate X. fig. 1.) The leap over the cord is made from the side of the stand towards which the heads of the pegs are turned; so that, if the feet touch the cord, it will easily and instantly fall.

In all kinds of leaping, it is of great importance to draw in and retain the breath at the moment of the greatest effort, as it gives the chest more solidity to support the rest of the members, impels the blood into the muscular parts, and increases their strength. The hands, also, should be shut, and the arms pendent. The extent of the leap in height, or horizontally, is proportioned to the power employed, and the practice acquired. As it is performed

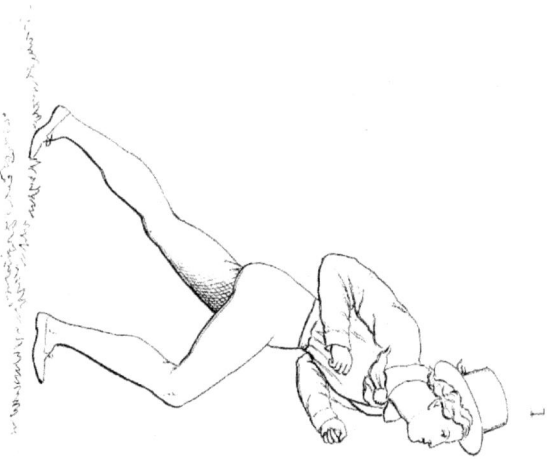

1

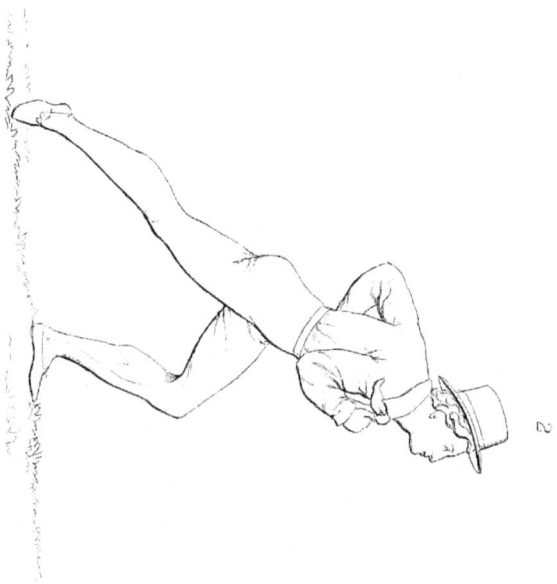

2

with facility only in proportion to the strength exerted, and the elasticity and suppleness of the articulations and muscles of the lower extremities, much exercise is necessary to attain that degree of perfection which lessens all obstacles, and supplies the means of clearing them without danger. Lightness and firmness are the qualities necessary for leaping: every thing should be done to acquire these two qualifications, for without them leaping is neither graceful nor safe.

THE HIGH LEAP.

Without a Run.

In this, the legs and feet are closed; the knees are bent till the calves nearly touch the thighs; the upper part of the body, kept straight, is inclined a little forward; and the arms thrown in the direction of the leap, which increases the impulse, preserves the balance, and may be useful in a fall. (Plate X. fig. 1.)

The vertebral column, and consequently the whole of the trunk, being thus bent forward, a strong contraction of the muscles preserves this bending till the moment when the leap takes place; then, by sudden contraction of the extensors, the body stretches out like a bow when the string breaks, is thus jerked forward, and remains suspended a longer or shorter time in the air.

In descending, the person should be rather inclined forward; and the fall should take place on the fore part of the feet, bending the knees and haunches, to deaden the shock and descent; for, the direct descent in this leap, if not thus broken, would send its shock from the heels to the spine and head, and might occasion injury. To perpen-

6

dicularity in this leap, should be added lightness, so that scarcely any noise from the leap should be heard.

This leap, without a run, may be practiced at the height,—

1. Of the knees.	3. Of the hips.
2. Of the middle of the thighs.	4. Of the lower ribs.

With a Run.

The run preceding the leap should never exceed ten paces, the distance between the point of springing and the cord being equal to half the cord's height from the ground. The view of the leaper should be directed first to the spot whence he is to spring; and, the moment he has reached that, to the cord, accustoming himself to spring from either foot, and from both feet.

The instant the spring is made, or (if it be made with one foot) immediately after, the feet should be closed, and the knees drawn forcibly towards the chin. Throughout, flexibility and skill, not violent exertion, should be displayed. This leap, with a run, may be practiced at the height,—

1. Of the hips.	5. Of the chin.
2. Of the lower ribs.	6. Of the eyes.
3. Of the pit of the stomach.	7. Of the crown of the head.
4. Of the breast.	

Feats in High Leaping.

A good high leaper will clear five feet; a first-rate one, five and a half; and an extraordinary one, six feet. Ireland is mentioned as having cleared an extended cord at the height of fourteen feet. Another man, it is said, jumped to the height of seventeen feet, which was three times the height of his own body.*

* The author means, with the aid of a spring-board.—Ed. Fifth Edition.

THE LONG LEAP.

Without a Run.

This is generally performed upon straight firm ground, on which there are marks, or parallel lines, at equal distances. The first of these lines is the place to leap from. The leapers succeed each other, and clear a greater number of lines, according to their strength and skill. Here the feet are closed; the whole weight rests upon the balls of the toes; and the body is inclined forward. Both arms are then swung forward,—backward,—then drawn strongly forward,—and at the same instant the limbs, having been bent, are extended with the utmost possible force.

In performing this leap, the hands and body must be bent forward, especially at the end of the movement, when the leaper alights. On level ground twelve feet is a good standing leap; and fourteen is one of comparatively rare occurrence.

With a Run.

This leap is best executed with a run; and we have therefore dwelt less upon the former. Here, also, the body must be inclined forward.

The run should be made over a piece of firm, and not slippery ground, to the extent of ten, fifteen, or twenty paces; should consist of small steps, increasing in quickness as they approach the point of springing; and these should be so calculated as to bring upon the point that foot with which the leaper is accustomed to spring. The spring, as here implied, should be performed with one foot, and the arms thrown forcibly towards the place proposed to be reached. The height as well as the length of the leap, must be calculated; for the leap is shortened by not springing a proper height. (Plate X. fig. 2.)

In the descent, the feet are closed, the knees bent, the upper part of the body inclined forward, and the toes first touch the ground, at which moment, a light spring, and afterwards some short steps, are made, in order to avoid any sudden check. In a much extended leap, however, alighting on the toes is impossible. A sort of horizontal swing is then achieved, by which the leaper's head is little higher than his feet, and his whole figure is almost parallel with the ground; and, in this case, to alight on the toes is impossible. Care must here be taken not to throw the feet so much forward as to cause the leaper to fall backward at the moment of descent. The ground must be cleared, or the leap is imperfect and unfair.

This leap may be practiced at,—

> 1. Double the length of the body.
> 2. Twice and a half that length.
> 3. Three times that length.

Feats in Long Leaping.

On level ground, twenty feet is a first-rate leap; twenty-one is extraordinary; and twenty-two is very rarely accomplished.* With a run and a leap, on a slightly inclined plane, twenty-three feet have been done.

Of the various kinds of leaps, the first or simple leap, which is produced principally by the extension of the abdominal members, which impel the body either straight upwards, in the vertical leap, or obliquely upwards and forwards, in the horizontal or rather parabolic leap, requires,

---

* I have seen twenty-two feet covered forwards and backwards, by an Irish tailor.—Ed. Fifth Edition.

in addition to the contraction of the abdominal members, especially if the leap be executed with the feet close together, a violent action of the muscles of the abdomen, upper parts of the back, anterior parts of the loins, and of the thorax and shoulders.

THE DEEP LEAP.

This may be made either with or without the hands. In either way, to avoid the shock, the body must be kept in a bent position, and the fall be upon the balls of the toes. When the hands are used, the leaper places them in front of the feet; and during the descent, the weight of the body is checked by the former, and passes in a diminished state to the latter; so that the shock is obviated.

A flight of steps serves the purpose of this exercise. The leaper ascends a certain number; leaps from the side; gradually increases the number; and, by practicing progressively higher, finds it easy to leap from heights which at first appalled him. He afterwards combines the long and deep leaps. For this purpose, a rivulet, which has one bank high and the opposite one low, is very favorable. Children can easily take a leap of nine feet in descending.

THE DEEP LEAP BACKWARDS, FROM A REST ON THE HANDS.

This exercise is first performed from platforms of various heights, and from walls of various elevations. The object is to lessen the shock that the legs and body experience in reaching the ground at a depth of more than six or seven feet, and to diminish the distance if possible, at the same time that it diminishes the violence and velocity of the fall. All this is easily managed by observing the following rules. Suppose the pupil placed upon a platform of four or six

feet in height, he must first examine the place he is about
to leap to, so as to select the most favorable part, free from
stones and other obstacles. He will then approach the extremity of the platform, with his back towards it, and bend
his body, placing his hands in the position shown in Plate
X. fig. 3. Having taken up this position securely, he will
lean his head a little forward, raise his toes from the platform, and remain for an instant supported by the arms.
The body then begins to extend, and the legs to lengthen
downwards and backwards; the arms follow this movement, bend, and support the body by the hands, which
have a secure resting-place on the edge of the platform, as
in Plate X. fig. 4. This descending movement is executed
as slowly as possible: the arms stretch out to their utmost
length, till the body is sustained by the last phalanx of the
fingers or touches the ground with the feet. If it does
not reach the ground, the pupil drops gently down on the
tips of his toes, bends himself, and recovers his upright
position.

There is another mode of descending, when the last resting-place for the hands is the top of a counterfort, or prop
on a wall without a counterfort. This consists (see Plate
X. fig. 3) in seizing the last hold with the right hand for
instance, and in hanging firmly by that hand, whilst the
left, being at liberty, is lowered and pushes back the body
from the projecting stones in the walls, to prevent injury
in the descent. The impulse thus given is, however, very
trifling, and solely to avoid hurt, without increasing the
violence of the fall, which ought to be facilitated on reaching the ground by the rules already given. By these means,
the height of a wall is relatively diminished, for a man
who hangs suspended by his arms, has six feet less to drop
than he who has his feet where he might put his hands.

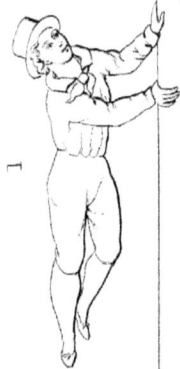

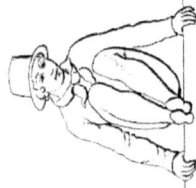

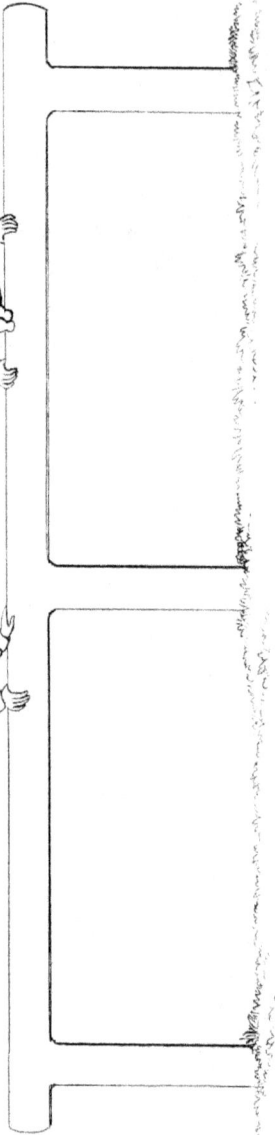

The down leap, unless gradually practiced, may produce rupture of the diaphragm. When, however, the elevation from which the leap is taken is gradually increased, the eye becomes accustomed to measure the most extensive distances fearlessly, at the same time that by practice the abdominal members learn to bend properly under the weight of the trunk, and thereby preserve the organs contained in it from serious injuries. In this kind of leap, the shocks will be diminished by retaining the air in the chest, which may be done by closing the glottis.

Persons who have long toes, powerful calves, and prominent heels, are the best adapted for leaping.

VAULTING.

In vaulting, by a spring of the feet, the body is raised, and by leaning the hands upon a fixed object, it at the same time receives, in oblique vaulting, a swing which facilitates the action. As the inclination thus given to the body depends not merely on the feet, but on the hands, we have the power to guide the body in any direction.

This exercise is conveniently practiced on the vaulting bar, which rests upon two or three posts. It may be performed with or without running. The beginner may at first be allowed a run of a few paces, ending in a preparatory spring; and he may afterwards be allowed only a spring.

OBLIQUE VAULTING.

To mount, the vaulter must place himself in front of the bar; make a preparatory spring with the feet close; fix at

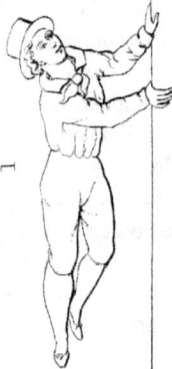

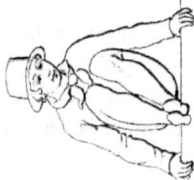

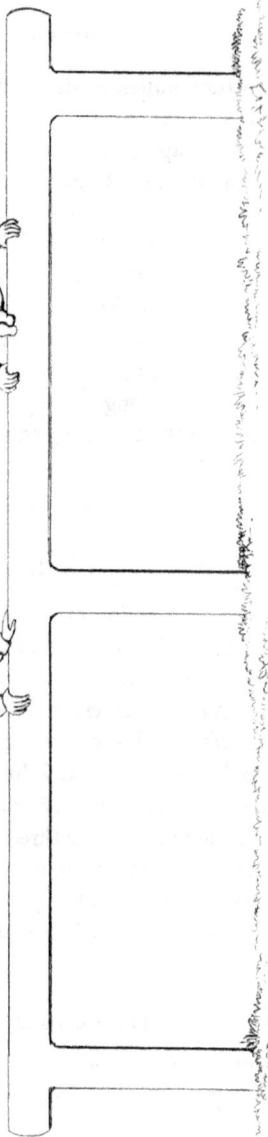

The down leap, unless gradually practiced, may produce rupture of the diaphragm. When, however, the elevation from which the leap is taken is gradually increased, the eye becomes accustomed to measure the most extensive distances fearlessly, at the same time that by practice the abdominal members learn to bend properly under the weight of the trunk, and thereby preserve the organs contained in it from serious injuries. In this kind of leap, the shocks will be diminished by retaining the air in the chest, which may be done by closing the glottis.

Persons who have long toes, powerful calves, and prominent heels, are the best adapted for leaping.

VAULTING.

In vaulting, by a spring of the feet, the body is raised, and by leaning the hands upon a fixed object, it at the same time receives, in oblique vaulting, a swing which facilitates the action. As the inclination thus given to the body depends not merely on the feet, but on the hands, we have the power to guide the body in any direction.

This exercise is conveniently practiced on the vaulting bar, which rests upon two or three posts. It may be performed with or without running. The beginner may at first be allowed a run of a few paces, ending in a preparatory spring; and he may afterwards be allowed only a spring.

OBLIQUE VAULTING.

To mount, the vaulter must place himself in front of the bar; make a preparatory spring with the feet close; fix at that moment both hands upon the bar; heave himself up, and swing the right leg over. The body, supported by the hands, may then easily descend into the riding position. To dismount, the vaulter, supported by the hands, must extend the feet, make a little swing forward, and a greater one backward, so as to heave both feet behind over the bar, and spring to the ground with them close.

To do this he must first clearly define to himself the place where he intends to fall. Then, having placed both hands upon the bar, he should first bend and then extend the joints, so as to raise the body with all his strength, and throw his legs, kept close, high over the bar. (Plate XI. fig. 1.) When the right hand (if he vault to the right) quits the bar, the left remains, the feet reach the ground on the opposite side, and he falls on both feet, with the knees projected, and the hands ready, if necessary, to break the fall.

In vaulting to the right, the left foot passes in the space which was between both hands, the right hand quits the bar, and the left guides the body in the descent. In vaulting to the left, the right foot passes in the space which was between both hands, the left hand quits the bar, and the right guides the body in its descent. As, however, it is difficult for beginners to vault either way, this is not to be attempted until after sufficient practice in the way which may be easiest. The vaulter may then, with a preparatory spring, try the following heights,—

    1. That of the pit of the stomach.

    2. That of a middling-sized horse.

    3. His own height or more.

STRAIGHT-FORWARD VAULTING.

For this purpose, both hands must be placed at such

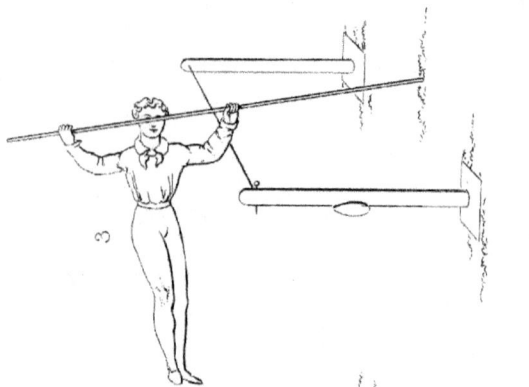

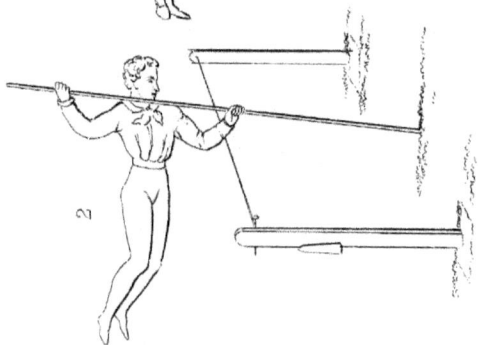

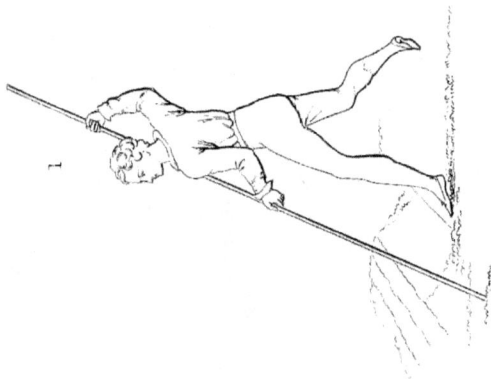

distance on the bar as to give room for the feet between them; the body should be forcibly raised; the knees drawn up towards the breast; and the feet brought between the hands, without moving them from their place. (Plate XI. fig. 2.) This should be practised until it can be done easily.

This straight-forward vault may have three different terminations. When the feet are in the space between the hands, the vaulter may stand upright. He may pass his feet to the opposite side, whilst he seats himself. He may continue to leap over the seat, through the arms, letting both hands go at once after the legs have passed.

LEAPING WITH A POLE.

This is a union of leaping and vaulting, in which the vaulter, instead of supporting himself upon a fixed object, carries with him a pole, which he applies to whatever spot he chooses. In supporting the body by a pole during the leap, a great deal also depends upon balancing, as well as on the strength of the arms and legs.

THE HIGH LEAP WITH A POLE.

The pole prescribed for this exercise is the planed stem of a straight-grown fir, from seven to ten feet long, and about two inches thick at the bottom. Such a pole naturally diminishes towards the top; and it is better to plane off the lower end a little. Care must be taken that it be sufficiently strong; such as make a crackling noise during the leap should be immediately thrown aside.

The learner, supposed to be already expert in leaping and

vaulting, may at first place himself before a small ditch, with a pole, which he holds in such a manner, that the right hand be about the height of the head, and the left about that of the hips, and in this case he must fix it in the ditch. (See Plate XII. fig. 1.) He must then, by making a spring with his left foot, endeavor to rest the weight of his body upon the pole, and, thus supported, swing himself to the opposite bank. In this swing, he passes his body by the right of the pole, making, at the same time, a turn, so that, at the descent, his face is directed to the place whence he leaped. The faults usually committed by the beginner, consist in his trusting to the pole the whole weight of the body; and in losing the necessary purchase by keeping at too great a distance from it.

This leap cannot be made with proper force and facility unless the fixing of the pole in the ground and the spring are made exactly at the same moment. To acquire this, the learner should place himself at the distance of a moderate pace in front of the ditch; raise the left foot and the pole together; plant both together, the former in the spot whence he intends making the spring, and the latter in the ditch; then instantly swing himself round the pole, to the opposite bank. As soon as he can easily take the proper position and balance, he may endeavor to swing his legs higher; and in proportion as he becomes more expert, he must place his hands higher up the pole, in order to have a greater swing. He must afterwards make a previous run of two, three, or four paces, gradually increasing in velocity; and always taking care that the springing foot and the pole come to the ground at the same moment. When this difficulty is overcome, he may practise the exercise over the leaping-stand.

In leaping over the cord, the learner must take the pole

in both hands; make a rather quick turn: conclude this
with the spring, and planting the pole at the same moment,
raise rapidly his whole body, by means of this spring and
a powerful support on the pole, and swing over the cord;
turning his body so that, at the descent, his face is directed
to the place whence he sprung. This is a general description of the high leap; but it is necessary to explain the
parts into which it may be divided, as follows,—

1. In the handling the pole (Plate XII. fig. 1,) it is immaterial, as to the lower hand, whether the thumb or the
little finger be uppermost: the upper hand must have the
thumb upward. The position of the upper hand is regulated by that of the lower one : as this advances higher up,
the former must be proportionally raised. The lower hand
then must be placed at a height proportionate to that of the
leap : thus, if the latter be six feet, the lower hand must
be at least from five and a half to six feet from the lower
end of the pole. The leaper is, after a little practice, enabled to seize the pole in the proper way, from a mere glance
at the leap.

2. The preparatory run of from twelve to fifteen paces is
accelerated as the leaper approaches the chord. Upon this
run principally depend the facility and the success of the
leap. As the spring can take place only with one foot, and
as this must arrive correctly at the springing place, it is
necessary that the order of the steps should be arranged so
as to effect this object. If the leaper should be obliged to
correct himself by making a few steps, either longer or
shorter, just before making the spring, the leap is rendered
difficult.

3. The fixing of the pole in the ground, and the spring,
must take place at the same instant, because by that means
the upper and lower members operate together, no power

is lost, and the swing is performed with the greatest facility. The place of the pole, however, varies with the height of the leaps; in leaps of about four feet, the distance of one foot from the cord is sufficient; in higher leaps, it should be from one and a half to two feet. The best plan is to have a small pit dug in front of the cord (see Plate XII. figs. 2 and 3,) and to remove the stand from it, as the height of the leap increases; or the stand may remain at a foot and a half from the pit, and the learner be taught to make all the leaps from it. The spring is made with one foot, at the distance of two, three, four, or five feet from the plant of the pole. If the leaper keep the left hand lowest, he must spring with the left foot, and *vice versa*.

4. The swing upward is effected by the force of the spring, the support of the lower, and the pull of the upper hand; but principally by the propulsion of the run, which being suddenly modified by the fixing of the pole, has its horizontal direction changed into a slanting ascent, and carries the body of the leaper over the cord. The leaper must carefully observe that the spring of the foot, and the plant of the pole, be in the direction of the preparatory run.

5. The turning of the body during the swinging upward, is necessary. When the leaper is going to spring, he has his face turned towards the object of the leap, as in Plate XVII. fig. 1; but as his feet swing, his body turns round the pole. When his feet have passed over the other side of the chord, the head is still considerably on this side: the leaper then appears as in fig. 2. Speedily, the middle of his body is on the other side of the cord, and he begins the descent, as in fig. 3. It would be impossible to descend in this position otherwise than with his face directed to the place where the leap was commenced.

6. The quitting of the pole during the leap is effected

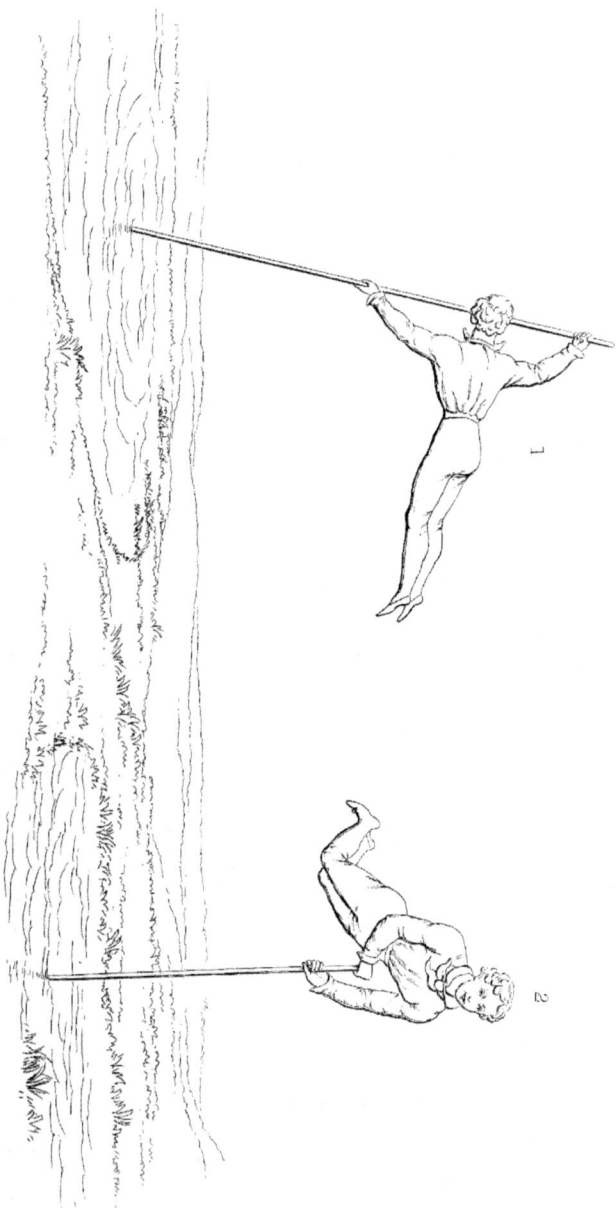

1

2

by giving it a push with one hand, at the moment of greatest height, and this causes it to fall on the inner side of the cord.

7. The carrying of the pole over the cord is more difficult. The leaper must then raise the pole a little from the ground at the moment of beginning the descent, and instantly elevate the lower part of it with the lowest hand, and depress the upper part with the other; the consequence being, that, at the descent, the lower end of the pole will point upward, and the upper end downward. This should be practised first in low leaps.

8. The descent depends entirely upon the manner in which the leap is made: if the leap be perfect, the descent will be so. The usual fault in descending is, that the leaper, having passed the cord, falls to the ground almost perpendicularly instead of obliquely. In the annexed figure, *a* is the place whence the spring is made, *c* the section of the cord, *b* the position of the leaper over it, *d* his right,

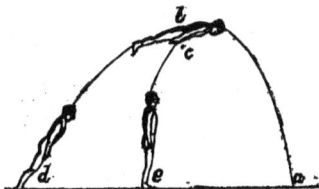

and *e* his wrong descent. The latter is faulty because it throws him so much out of balance, that in order not to fall backward, he must run backward to *d*. If, on the contrary, he descends in proper balance to the ground, he moves not an inch from the spot where his feet alight; and this complete rest following the descent is the sign of a

7

perfect leap. The descent, as already explained, must take place upon the balls of the toes, and with a sinking of the knees. The position of the body is sufficiently explained by Plate XII. figs. 1, 2, and 3; but many learn to swing the legs so well as to raise them, during the highest part of the leap, considerably above the head. Order of exercises in the high leap, to be very gradually attempted :—

1. The height of the hips.
2. That of the pit of the stomach.
3. That of the chin.

4. That of the crown of the head.
5. That of the points of the fingers—that is, as high as the latter can reach.

In performing these leaps, the pole is parted with. As many more may form a repetition of the preceding, with this difference, that the leaper carries the pole over with him. A similar number may repeat the first, except that the leaper, between the spring and descent, makes a complete turn round the pole, so as again to bring his face in the direction of the leap. This enlarged turn is rendered easier by leaping a little higher than the cord requires.

THE LONG LEAP WITH A POLE.

This leap is the most useful, being applicable almost everywhere; and particularly in a country intersected with small rivers, ditches, &c. It should be first practised over a ditch about three feet deep, eight feet broad at one end, and about twenty-one feet at the other, and of any convenient length. In this exercise, the pole should be rather stronger and longer than in the preceding one—depending, however, on the length of the leap, and the height of the bank it is made from. The usual length is from ten to thirteen feet.

The handling of the pole is the same as in the high leap.

The preparatory run is rapid, in proportion to the length of the leap. The spring takes place as in the preceding exercise. The swing is also the same, except that the curve of the leap is wider. The turning of the body may likewise be similar, but it is convenient to make only a quarter turn. In the descent, the hand presses more upon the pole; and the feet are stretched out to reach the opposite bank, as in Plate XIII. fig. 1, in which the leaper is descending. Another method of leaping a river, is to force the body up so high by the pressure of the hands (of which one rests upon the end of the pole, or very near it,) as to swing over the top of the pole, and allow it to pass between the legs when descending. (Plate XII. fig. 2.)

Try the following :—

1. The leap of two lengths of the body.	3. That of four lengths of the body.
2. That of three lengths of the body.	4. Persons of equal strength try to outleap one another.

The lengths of 18, 20, 22, and 24 feet are frequently done by practised leapers.

THE DEEP LEAP WITH A POLE.

Here neither the preparatory run nor the spring occur : there is nothing which requires the exertion of the lower members. The use of the hands and arms, however, is peculiarly requisite, as well as a little of the art of balancing. The leaper fixes the pole, at a convenient distance from the place where he stands, in a chasm, ditch, or river, having one bank high, and the opposite one low. Seizing it with both hands in the usual way, he slips along it lower and lower; the whole weight of his body, at last, resting upon it. Thus, if the depth is considerable, as two lengths of the body, he may slide so far down upon it, that his head appears slanting downward. In this position, he makes a slight push against the bank, or merely quits it, with his feet, which he swings by the side of the pole to the opposite bank. Here, also, the descent is performed upon the balls of the toes, with bending of the knees. The principal advantage in this leap lies in the art of supporting the body, without tottering; and for this purpose, it is absolutely necessary that the feet should be stretched out far from each other, in an angular form, otherwise the balance might be lost. The best way of practising this in an exercise ground, is by a flight of steps.

To the exercise of the abdominal members, these leaps unite a strong action of the muscles of the thorax, arms, and forearms, and even of those of the palms of the hand. The body is only half impelled by the abdominal members; but this impulse is rendered complete by considerable effort on the part of the thoracic members. The latter, in the vertical leap, being supported by the narrow and moveable base afforded by the pole, assist greatly in raising the body, and even keep it a moment suspended for the legs to pass over (if the object to be cleared is very high) before it allows the body to obey the force of gravity which carries it down.

This exercise communicates what is termed great lightness to the body, and great suppleness—that is to say, great relative strength of the abdominal members; and it also developes the superior members. It is good for lymphatic temperaments and young persons, but it should not be indulged in immediately after meals. It may occasion accidents of the brain and spinal marrow, unless all the articulations are bent on returning to the ground.

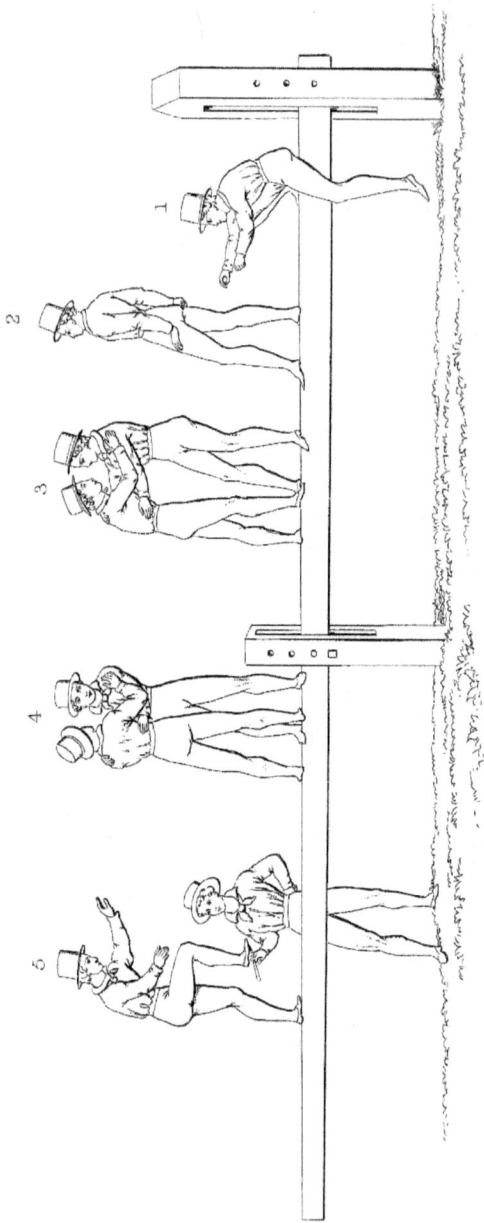

BALANCING.

Balancing is the art of preserving the stability of the body upon a narrow or a moving surface. The balancing bar consists of a round and tapering pole, supported horizontally, about three feet from the ground, by upright posts, one at its thicker extremity, and another about the middle, between the parts of which it may be raised or lowered by means of an iron peg passing through holes in their sides. The unsupported end of the bar wavers, of course, when stepped upon—(Plate XIV.)

The upper surface of the bar being smooth in dry weather, the soles of the shoes should be damped; the ground about the bar should consist of sand, and the exercises be cautiously performed.

POSITION AND ACTION IN BALANCING.

In this exercise, the head should be held up, the body erect, the shoulders back, the arms extended, the hands shut, and the feet turned outwards. At first, the balancer may be assisted along the bar; but he must gradually receive less and less aid, till at last the assistant only remains by his side.

The pole may be mounted either from the ground or from the riding position on the beam. In the latter case, the balancer may raise the right foot, place it flat on the beam, with the heel near the upper part of the thigh, and rise on the point of the foot, carrying the weight of the body before him. (Plate XIV. fig. 1.)

In this case, the beam must not be touched with the hands; the left leg must hang perpendicularly, with the toe towards the ground, and the arms be stretched forward.

7*

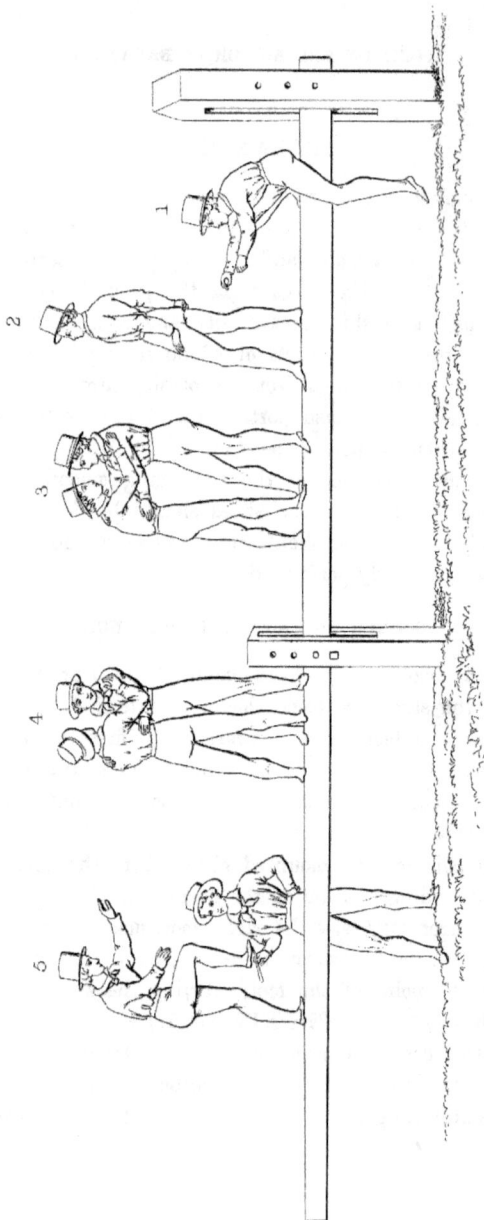

BALANCING.

Balancing is the art of preserving the stability of the body upon a narrow or a moving surface. The balancing bar consists of a round and tapering pole, supported horizontally, about three feet from the ground, by upright posts, one at its thicker extremity, and another about the middle, between the parts of which it may be raised or lowered by means of an iron peg passing through holes in their sides. The unsupported end of the bar wavers, of course, when stepped upon—(Plate XIV.)

The upper surface of the bar being smooth in dry weather, the soles of the shoes should be damped; the ground about the bar should consist of sand, and the exercises be cautiously performed.

POSITION AND ACTION IN BALANCING.

In this exercise, the head should be held up, the body erect, the shoulders back, the arms extended, the hands shut, and the feet turned outwards. At first, the balancer may be assisted along the bar; but he must gradually receive less and less aid, till at last the assistant only remains by his side.

The pole may be mounted either from the ground or from the riding position on the beam. In the latter case, the balancer may raise the right foot, place it flat on the beam, with the heel near the upper part of the thigh, and rise on the point of the foot, carrying the weight of the body before him. (Plate XIV. fig. 1.)

In this case, the beam must not be touched with the hands; the left leg must hang perpendicularly, with the toe towards the ground, and the arms be stretched forward.

After keeping the balance for some minutes in this position, he must stretch the left leg out before him, place his heel on the middle of the beam, with the toe well turned outward, and transfer the weight of the body from the point of the right foot to the left heel—(Plate XIV. fig. 2.) These steps he must perform alternately, till he reaches the end of the beam.

TURNS IN BALANCING.

When the balancer is able to walk firmly and in good position along the bar, and to spring off whenever he may lose his balance, he may attempt to turn round, first at the broad, then at the narrow end, and to return. He may next try to go backward.

In accomplishing this, it is no longer the heel, but the tip of the toes, which receives the weight; the leg which hangs being stretched backward, with the hip, knee, and heel forming a right angle, till the toes, by a transverse motion, are so placed on the middle of the beam, that the balancer can safely transfer to them the whole weight of the body.

To acquire the art of passing an obstacle placed laterally, two balancers may pass each other thus :—They must hold one another fast by the arms, advance breast to breast, place each his right foot close forward to that of his comrade, across the bar, (Plate XIV. fig. 3,) and turn completely round each other, by each stepping with his left foot round the right one of the other, as in Plate XIV. fig. 4.

To acquire the art of passing an obstacle placed inferiorly, a large stone may be laid upon the bar, or a stick may be held before the balancer, about the height of the knee. (Plate XIV. fig. 5.)

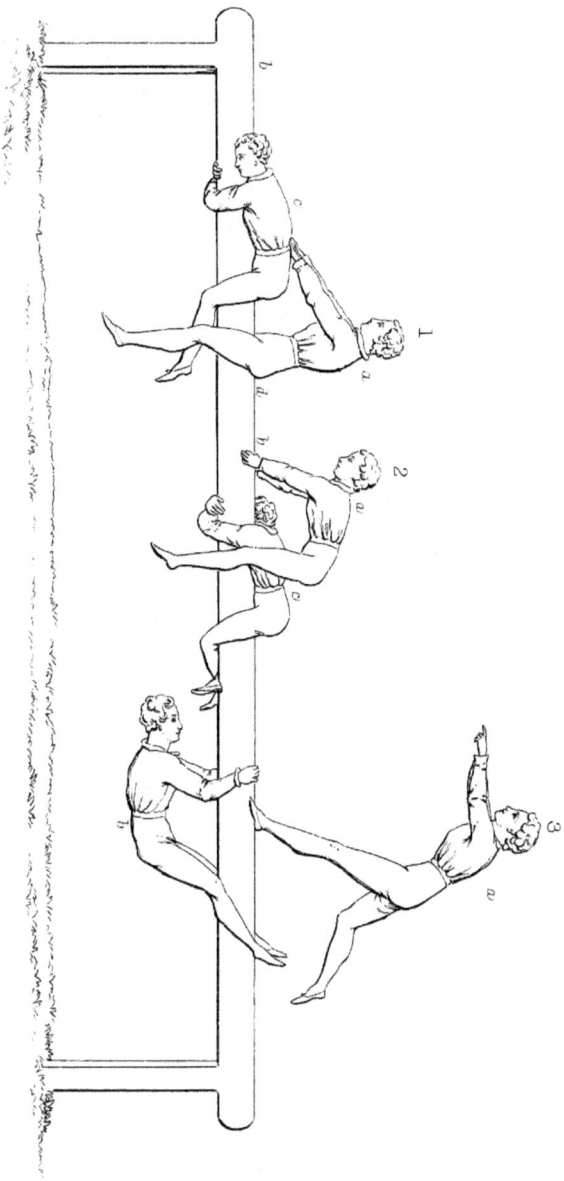

To pass over men placed upon a beam, the pupil or pupils who are astride in front lie down on the beam, which they grasp firmly by passing their arms round it. The pupil *a* (fig. 1, Plate XX.) having to pass to the point on the beam marked *b*, places his hands on the waistband of his comrade *c* : he then leans upon his arms, and raises his body to pass forward over his comrade, opening his legs widely, so as not to touch him, till he places himself astride at *c*. He then extends his hands and arms for a second movement, places them at *b*, and leans the body well forward, as shown in fig. 2, Plate XV. Being thus placed, he makes the last movement, raises his body upon the arms to pass over his comrade's head without touching it, which is the chief rule of this exercise, and places himself astride upon the beam at *b*, moving his hands immediately, and extending them to rest at *d*. This movement being finished, he continues advancing astride, along the beam, over the others, if there be any; raises himself to an upright position, and lies down in his turn on the beam. This last attitude requires some care, because the head must incline either to the right or left of the beam, as shown in the plates, and the pupil must hold tight to the beam with the arms and thighs, which requires both skill and strength.

The pupil may also pass as shown in fig. 3, Plate XV. This method is very easy for the person passing and indeed more so than any other; but it is necessary that the pupil who is in the position *b* should have learnt to raise himself up on the beam, or know how to advance along it underneath, in a reversed position.

It is impossible for any one who has not seen the carnivals of Venice, and other towns in Italy, to form an idea of all the difficulties that have been surmounted in the art of equilibrium. To acquire the art of carrying any body, the balancer may at first walk along the bar with his hands folded across his breast, instead of using them to balance himself; and he may afterwards carry bodies of various magnitudes.

To this notice of the rules by which the art of Balancing may be best acquired, it will not be out of place to subjoin a slight outline of its importance to all who desire to arrive at excellence in any of the Manly Exercises. Motion— the source of them all—if not absolutely dependent for existence upon equilibrium, without it would be but the infancy of action—movement tottering, uncertain, powerless. The first effort of locomotion—the walk, without it, possesses neither force nor decision : in the same ratio that a higher degree of muscular exertion is demanded, increases the value and importance of the art which teaches how best to apply the vital energies to its service. What a wise economy is to the social, this art is to the physical system : both serve to augment our resources, by instructing us so to husband them that the term " necessity " be not known to our vocabulary.

While in every instance equilibrium adds greatly to physical power, in many it stands altogether in its stead. To the most casual observer of our usual sports it will be manifest that this is the case in Skating ;—the more attentive and competent will have little difficulty in tracing its effects in Leaping, Vaulting, Swimming, and through almost the whole catalogue. It is to the later writers on horsemanship that we are indebted for the knowledge of its vital service to the equestrian. The truth of their theory is proved by the fact that, where formerly scarce a

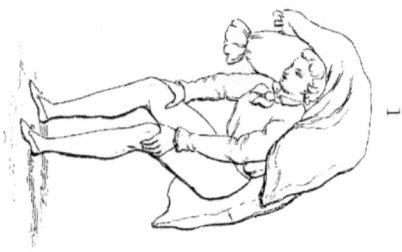

1

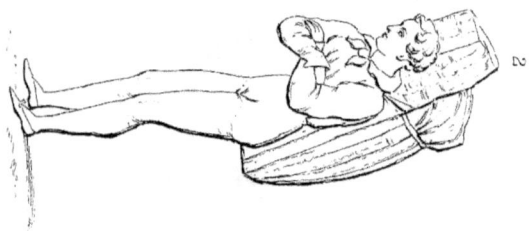

2

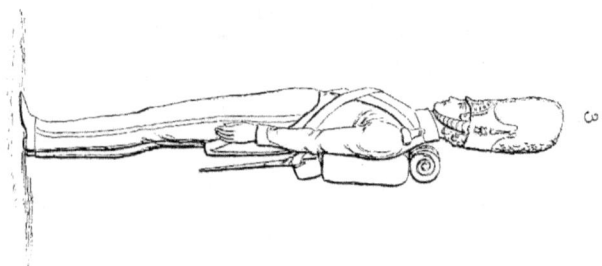

3

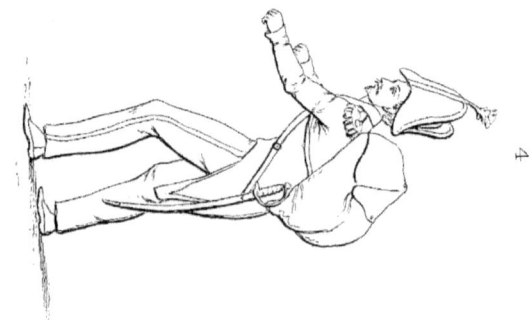

4

tithe of a hunting-field was found to ride to hounds, now nine-tenths are ordinarily to be seen in good places.

—————— Scouring along,
In pleasing hurry and confusion toss'd,
Happy the man, who with unrival'd speed
Can pass his fellows.

CARRYING WEIGHT.

The power of raising and carrying weight is of great importance in a general view. Many advantages will be derived from it; for besides strengthening the locomotive muscles, upon which all our physical operations depend, it will fortify also all the system and all the organs. All persons, moreover, may find themselves under the necessity of raising and carrying a wounded or fainting person, and may be glad to have cultivated and acquired the power necessary to perform such an act.

In accustoming young persons to carry burdens, they should be taught to support what is on the back first with one hand and then with the other; by these means the muscles are equally exercised on each side, and acquire an equal development. These burdens, however, must not exceed their strength; and they should be taught not to carry on one side in preference, for fear of deforming the limbs. There are several modes of supporting weights, and of trying the amount of power possessed for this kind of exercise.

Fig. 1, Plate XVII. represents one method. It consists in loading the shoulders with sacks full of articles whose weight is previously known. The position of the arms and hands such that the pupil can support a great weight : but in this way he can walk but very slowly; and it is therefore, so far, disadvantageous.

Fig. 2, in the same plate, supports a weight by means of a hod. This is filled with balls or stones, of which the weight is known.

The form of the weight is of consequence. A soldier now carries with ease a knapsack full of articles, and additional weight above it, because the flat shape that has been lately adopted fits the body, and lies close to the back, as in fig. 3, and the centre of gravity is thus very little deranged. But if the knapsack were of the old shape, very projecting and very round, as in fig. 4, the soldier would be forced to incline his body forward, and would not be able to carry as great a weight, nor march as long a time, in consequence of fatigue. It is for this reason, among others, desirable to extend the knowledge of the most simple rules of mechanics, because these rules are serviceable in avoiding many dangers, and diminishing the fatigue and the efforts that vacillation in the movements produces. We may make use of a hook to bear boxes or bags in addition, with the weights marked, and thus learn the carrier's strength.

Milo, says history, first carried a calf immediately after its birth, and continued to do so every day till it had reached its full size. It was said by this means that he was able to carry even the ox itself, and afterwards throw it on the ground and kill it with his fist.

Augustus the Second, King of Poland, carried a man upon his hand.

A man named Roussel, a labourer in the environs of Lisle, who on a smaller scale (being but four feet ten inches in height), was formed exactly like the Farnese

Hercules, raised on his shoulders a weight of eighteen hundred pounds. He cleared a circle six feet in height with very little spring and one hundred weight in each hand. When seated on the ground, he rose up without aid, carrying two men on his arms. Equally astonishing in the strength of his loins, he took up two hundred-weight leaning backwards over a chair. "I have seen this remarkable man," says Friedlander: "the whole of his family are very strong: his sister and brother are equally remarkable in this point." It is very striking to find in him the characteristic traits with which antiquity depicted the ideal of bodily strength.

In the Encyclopædia of Kruntz, vol. lxxii., we find instances of some men similar to Roussel, who lived at the commencement of the last century. A man named Eckenberg raised a cannon of two thousand five hundred pounds weight; and two strong men were unable to take from him a stick that he held between his teeth.

In number 446 of the Bibliotheque Britannique, is to be found a report of some trials made by a Mr. Shulze, in his manufactory, of the strength of men of different heights. These trials show what influence an elevated stature has upon the vertical height to which a man can raise any weight. A short man is, in his turn, capable of employing more force in another direction.

THROWING THE DISCUS.

Among the Greeks, throwing the discus did not form part of the games till the eighteenth Olympiad. This exercise consisted in throwing, as far as possible, a mass of wood or stone, but more commonly of iron or copper, of a lenticular form. From the testimony of ancient authors, there was no mark or butt fixed, except the spot where the discus thrown by the strongest of the discoboli alighted. Mercuriali has handed down to us three engravings, in which the discus is not of the same shape. The first engraving represents four discoboli in the act of throwing with the right hand a discus which is as thick at the circumference as at the centre, which has been bored. The second represents the statue of a discobulus holding a discus apparently of a spherical form, in the left hand. The third shows the arm of an athlete with a flat discus. The discus in the last two engravings now mentioned, covers the greater part of the front of the forearm; and all that the ancients have written respecting this instrument, tends to show that it was of enormous size and weight. Homer tells us, that the athletes threw the discus either up into the air merely as a prelude to accustom their arms to it, or horizontally when they were striving for the prize.

To perform this exercise properly, the thrower should not only balance the discus well on the right arm, (supposing it to be on that arm, as in Plate XVII. fig. 1;) but at the moment it leaves the hand, he should throw the whole of the right side forward, so that the impulse may be assisted by the weight of the whole body. (Plate XVII. fig. 2.) This exercise very much strengthens the body, and developes, in a particular manner, the limb by which the discus is thrown. It may be usefully employed in cases where it is desirable to remedy weakness in either of the arms; and it is well calculated to bring up the power of the left arm to that of the right. The modern quoit differs from the ancient discus only in this, that the instrument so called is much smaller than the discus, that its use is a mere idle

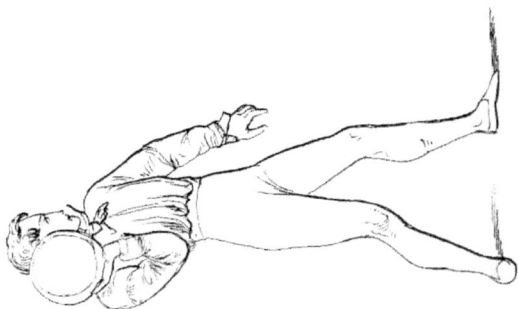

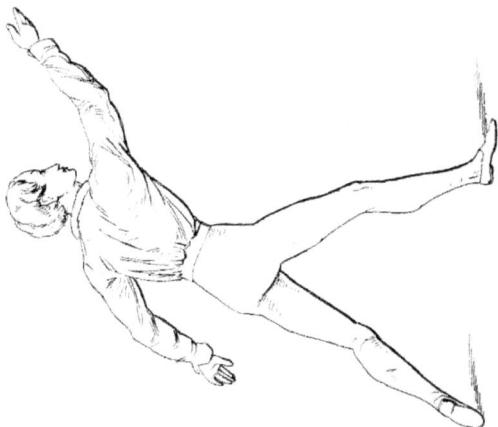

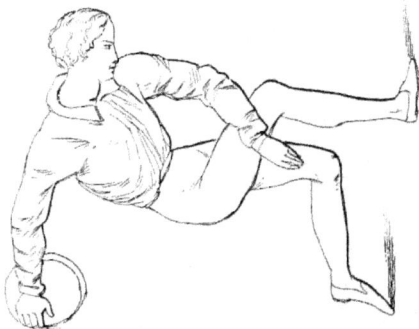

pastime, and that the object is always to throw it as close as possible to a fixed mark, requiring more skill than strength.

It is evident that the discus may be heaved from above the shoulder as well as flung from below.—(See Plate XVII. fig. 3.) No exercises can excel these for the acquirement of power. They ought to be much practised with both hands. A man of moderate strength will throw a pound weight of lead a distance of 140 feet, or thereabouts.

Silex 1½	.	.	.	126 feet.
Ditto ¼	.	.	.	145 "
Brick ½	.	.	.	160 "

CLIMBING.

Climbing is the art of transporting the body in any direction, by the aid, in general, both of the hands and feet. The climbing-stand consists of two strong poles, about fifteen feet high, and from fifteen to twenty-five feet distant, which are firmly fixed on the ground, and support a beam strongly fastened to them. One pole is two inches and a half in diameter; the other, which serves as a mast, should be considerably thicker; and both serve the purpose of climbing. To the beam are attached other implements of climbing: viz. a ladder, an inclined board, a mast, an inclined pole, a horizontal bar, a rope ladder, an upright, an inclined, and a level rope.—(Plate XVIII.)

KINDS OF CLIMBING. •

Climbing on fixed bodies should first be practised.

The Ladder.

Exercises on the ladder may be practised in the following ways:—

1. By ascending and descending as usual.

2. With one hand, carrying something in the other.

3. Without using the hands.

4. Passing another on the front of the ladder, or swinging to the back, to let another pass.

The Inclined Board.

This should be rather rough, about two feet broad, and two inches thick. To climb it, it is necessary to seize both sides with the hands, and to place the feet flat in the middle, the inclination of the board being diminished with the progress of the pupil.

At first, it may form with the ground an angle of about thirty degrees; and the climber should not go more than half-way up. This angle may gradually be augmented to a right angle, or the direction of the board may be made perpendicular. When the board is thus little or not at all inclined, the body must be much curved inward, and the legs thrust up, so that the higher one is nearly even with the hand. In descending, small and quick steps are necessary.

The Upright Pole.

The upright pole should be about two inches and a half in diameter, perfectly smooth and free from splinters.

The position of the climber is shown in Plate XVIII. fig. 1, where nothing touches the pole except the feet, legs, knees, and hands. He grasps as high as possible with both hands, raises himself by bending the body and drawing his legs up the pole, holds fast by them, extends the body, again grasps higher up with his hands, and continues the

same use of the legs and arms. The descent is performed
by sliding down with the legs, and scarcely touching with
the hands, as in Plate XVIII. fig. 2.

The Mast.

This is more difficult, as it cannot be grasped with the
hands; and it consequently should not be practised until
the climber is expert in the previous exercises. The position of the legs is the same as for the pole; but, instead of
grasping the mast, the climber lays hold of his left arm
with his right hand, or the reverse, and clings to the mast
with the whole body, as in Plate XVIII. fig. 3.

The Slant Pole.

This must be at least three inches thick; and as, in this
exercise, the hands bear more of the weight than in
climbing the upright pole, it should not be attempted until
expertness in the other is acquired.

The Horizontal, or Slightly Inclined Bar.

This may be about two inches wide at top, from ten to
fifteen feet long, and supported by two posts, respectively
six and seven feet high. The climber must grasp with both
hands as high a part of the bar as he can reach, and, with
arms extended, support his own weight as long as possible.
He must next endeavor to bend the elbows so much, that
one shoulder remains close under the bar, as seen in Plate
XVIII. fig. 4. Or he may place both hands on the same
side, and draw himself up so far as to see over it, keeping
the legs and feet close and extended.

He may then hang with his hands fixed on both sides,
near to each other, having the elbows much bent, the upper

parts of the arms close to the body, and one shoulder close under the bar; may lower the head backwards, and may, at the same time, raise the feet to touch each other over the bar.—(Plate XVIII. fig. 5.) In the last position, he may move the hands one before the other, forward or backward, and may either slide the feet along the bar, or alternately change them like the hands, and retain a similar hold.

Hanging also by the hands alone, as in Plate XVIII. fig. 6, he moves them either forward or backward, keeping the arms firm, and the feet close and extended. Or he may place himself in front of the bar, hanging by both hands, and move laterally. Being likewise in front of the bar, with his hands resting upon it, as in Plate XVIII. fig. 7, he may move along the bar either to the right or left. In the position of Plate XVIII. fig. 5, the climber may endeavor to sit upon the bar, for instance, on the right side, by taking hold with the right knee-joint, grasping firmly with the right hand, and bringing the left armpit over the bar. The riding position is thus easily obtained. From the riding position, he may, by supporting himself with one thigh, turn towards the front of the bar, allowing the leg of the other side to hang down; and he may then very easily move along the bar sideways, by raising his body with his hands placed laterally on the bar.

The Rope Ladder.

This should have several rundles to spread it out, and ought, in all respects, to be so constructed, as not to twist and entangle. The only difficulty here is that, as it hangs perpendicularly, and is flexible, its steps are liable to be pushed forward, and in that case, the body is thrown into an oblique position, and the whole weight falls on the

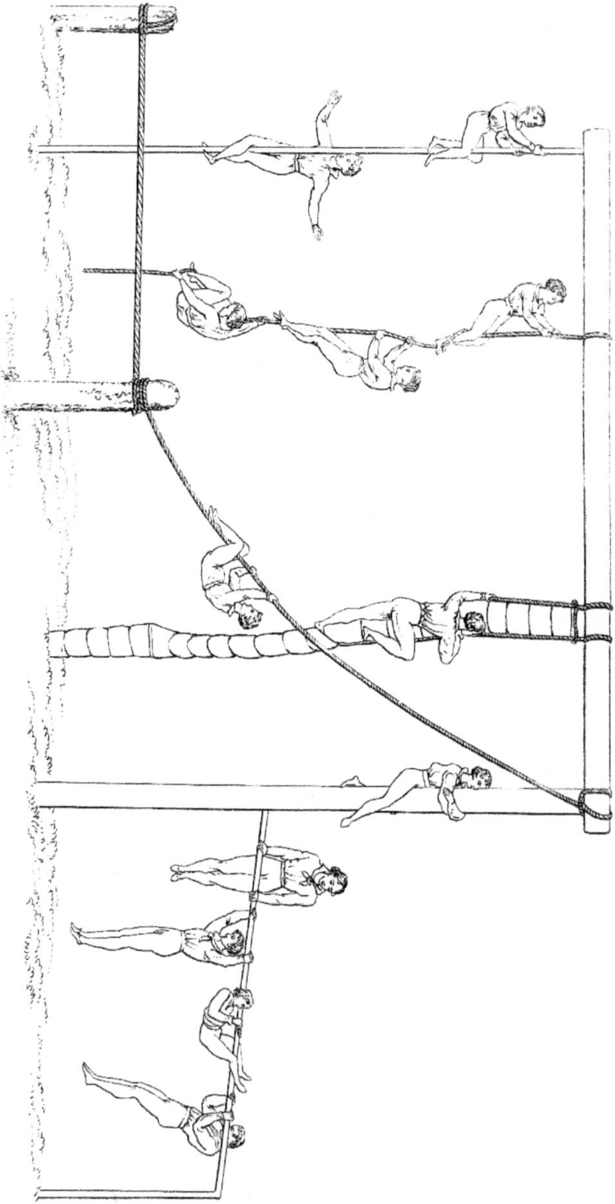

hands. To prevent this, the climber must keep the body stretched out and upright.—(Plate XVIII. fig. 8.)

The Upright Rope.

In this exercise, the securing the rope may be effected in various ways. In the first method, shown in Pl. XVIII. fig. 9. the hands and feet alone are employed. The feet are crossed; the rope passes between them, and is held fast by their pressure; the hands then grasp higher; the feet are drawn up; they are again applied to the rope; and the same process is repeated. In the second, which is the sailor's method, shown at Pl. XVIII. fig. 10, the rope passes from the hands, generally along the right thigh, just above the knee; winds round the inside of the thigh, under the knee-joint, over the outside of the leg, and across the instep, whence it hangs loose; and the climber, by treading with the left foot upon that part of the rope where it crosses the right one, is firmly supported. This mode of climbing requires the right leg and foot to be so managed that the rope keeps its proper winding whenever it is quitted by the left foot. In descending, to prevent injury, the hands must be lowered alternately.

To rest upon the upright rope, shown in Pl. XVIII. fig. 11, the climber must swing the right foot around the rope, so as to wind it three or four times round the leg; must turn it, by means of the left foot, once or twice round the right one, of which the toes are to be bent upwards; and must tread firmly with the left foot upon the last winding. Or, to obtain a more perfect rest he may lower his hands along the rope, as in Figure 11, hold with the right hand, stoop, grasp with the left the part of the rope below the feet, raise it and himself again, and wind it round his shoulders, &c., until he is firmly supported.

8*

The Oblique Rope.

The climber must fix himself to the rope, as in Pl. XVIII.
fig. 12, and advance the hands along it, as already directed.
The feet may move along the rope alternately; or one leg,
hanging over the rope, may slide along it; or, which is
best, the sole of one foot may be laid upon the rope, and
the other leg across its instep, so that the friction is not felt.

The Level Rope.

This may have its ends fastened to posts of equal heights;
and the same exercises may be performed upon it.

Climbing Trees.

In attempting this exercise, the kind of the wood and
strength of the branches must be considered. Summer is
the best time for practicing it, as withered branches are
then most easily discerned; and even then it is best to climb
low trees, until some experience is acquired. As the surface of branches is smooth, or moist and slippery, the hands
must never for a moment be relaxed.

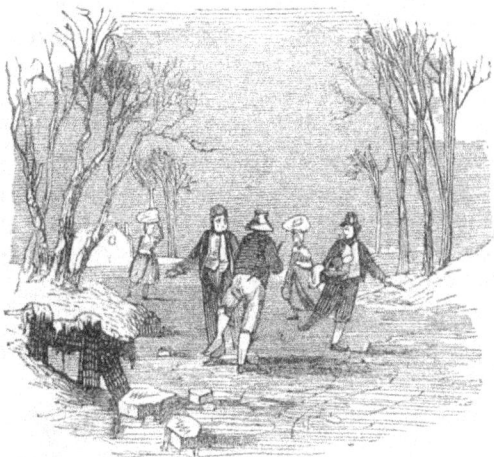

SKATING.

SKATING is the art of balancing the body, while, by the impulse of each foot alternately, it moves rapidly upon the ice.

CONSTRUCTION OF THE SKATE.

The wood of the skate should be slightly hollowed, so as to adapt it to the ball of the foot; and, as the heel of the boot must be thick enough to admit the peg, it may be well to lower the wood of the skate corresponding to the heel, so as to permit the foot to regain that degree of horizontal position which it would otherwise lose by the height of the heel; for the more of the foot that is in contact with the skate, the more firmly will these be attached. As the tread of the skate should correspond, as nearly as possible, with that of the foot, the wood should be of the same length as the boot or shoe; the irons of good steel, and well secured in the wood.

These should pass beyond the screw at the heel, nearly as far as the wood itself; but the bow of the iron should not project much beyond the tread.

If the skate project much beyond the wood, the whole foot, and more especially its hind part, must be raised considerably from the ice when the front or bow of the skate is brought to bear upon it; and, as the skater depends upon this part for the power of his stroke, it is evident that that must be greatly diminished by the general distance of the foot from the ice. In short, if the skate be too long, the stroke will be feeble, and the back of the leg painfully cramped: if it be too short, the footing will be proportionally unsteady and tottering.

As the position of the person in the act of skating is never vertical, and is some times very much inclined, and as considerable exertion of the muscles of the leg is requisite to keep the ankle stiff, this ought to be relieved by the lowness of the skates. Seeing, then, that the closer the foot is to the ice, the less is the strain on the ankle, it is clear that the foot ought to be brought as near to the ice as possible, without danger of bringing the sole of the shoe in contact with it, while traversing on the edge of the skate. The best height is about three-quarters of an inch, and the iron about a quarter of an inch thick.

The grooved or fluted skate, if ever useful, is of service only to boys, or very light persons, whose weight is not sufficient to catch the ice in a hard frost. It certainly should never be used by a person who is heavier than a boy of thirteen or fourteen years of age usually is, because the sharp edge too easily cuts into the ice, and prevents figuring. Fluted skates, indeed, are even dangerous: for the snow or ice cuttings are apt to collect and consolidate in the grooves, till the skater is raised from the edge of his skate, and thrown.

In the general inclination of the foot in skating, no edge can have greater power than that of rectangular shape : the tendency of its action is downwards, cutting through rather than sliding on the surface; and greater hold than this is unnecessary. The irons of skates should be kept well and sharply ground. This ought to be done across the stone, so as to give the bottom of the skate so slight a concavity as to be imperceptible, which insures an edge whose angle is not greater than right. Care must be taken that one edge is not higher than the other; so that when the skate is placed upon an even surface, it may stand quite perpendicularly. The wear of the iron not being great with a beginner, one grinding will generally last him through an ordinary winter's skating on clean ice.

The bottom of the iron should be a little curved; for, if perfectly straight, it would be capable of describing only a straight line, whereas the skater's progress must be circular, because, in order to bring the edge to bear, the body must be inclined, and inclination can be preserved only in circular motion. This curve of the iron should be part of a circle, whose radius is about two feet. That shape enables the skater to turn his toe or heel outwards or inwards with facility.

A screw would have a firmer hold than a mere peg in the hole of the boot; but, as it is less easily removed, skaters generally prefer the peg. The skater should be careful not to bore a larger hole in the heel than is sufficient to admit the peg. The more simple the fastenings of the skate the better. The two straps—namely, the cross strap over the toe, and the heel strap—cannot be improved, unless perhaps by passing one strap through the three bores, and so making it serve for both.

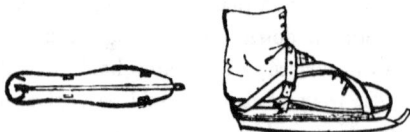

Before going on the ice, the young skater must learn to tie on the skates, and may also learn to walk with them easily in a room, balancing alternately on each foot.

DRESS OF THE SKATER.

A skater's dress should be as close and unincumbered as possible. Large skirts get entangled with his own limbs, or those of the persons who pass near him; and all fullness of dress is exposed to the wind. Loose trousers, frocks, and more especially great coats, must be avoided; and indeed, by wearing additional under-clothing, they can always be dispensed with.

As the exercise of skating produces perspiration, flannel next the chest, shoulders, and loins, is necessary to avoid the evils produced by sudden chills in cold weather. The best dress is what is called a dress-coat, buttoned, tight pantaloons, and laced boots (having the heel no higher than is necessary for the peg,) which hold the foot tightly and steadily in its place, as well as give the best support to the ankle; for it is of no use to draw the straps of the skate hard, if the boot or the shoe be loose.

PRELIMINARY AND GENERAL DIRECTIONS.

Either very rough or very smooth ice should be avoided. The person who for the first time attempts to skate, must not trust to a stick. He may make a friend's hand his

support, if he require one ; but that should be soon relin-
quished, in order to balance himself. He will probably
scramble about for half an hour or so, till he begins to find
out where the edge of his skate is.

The beginner must be fearless, but not violent; nor even
in a hurry. He should not let his feet get far apart, and
keep his heels still nearer together. He must keep the
ankle of the foot on the ice quite firm; not attempting to
gain the edge of the skate by bending it, because the right
mode of getting to either edge is by the inclination of the
whole body in the direction required; and this inclination
should be made fearlessly and decisively.

The leg which is on the ice should be kept perfectly
straight; for, though the knee must be somewhat bent at
the time of striking, it must be straightened as quickly as
possible without any jerk. The leg which is off the ice
should also be kept straight, though not stiff, having an easy
but slight play, the toe pointing downwards, and the heel
within from six to twelve inches of the other.

The learner must not look down at the ice, nor at his
feet, to see how they perform. He may at first incline his
body a little forward, for safety, but hold his head up, and
see where he goes, his person erect, and his face rather
elevated than otherwise.

When once off, he must bring both feet up together, and
strike again, as soon as he finds himself steady enough,
rarely allowing both feet to be on the ice together. The
position of the arms should be easy and varied; one being
always more raised than the other, this elevation being alternate, and the change corresponding with that of the
legs ; that is, the right arm being raised as the right leg is
put down, and *vice vesrâ*, so that the arm and leg of the
same side may not be raised together.

The face must be always turned in the direction of the line intended to be described. Hence, in backward skating, the head will be inclined much over the shoulder; in forward skating, but slightly. All sudden and violent action must be avoided. Stopping may be caused by slightly bending the knees, drawing the feet together, inclining the body forward, and pressing on the heels. It may also be caused by turning short to the right or left, the foot on the side to which we turn being rather more advanced, and supporting part of the weight.

THE ORDINARY RUN, OR INSIDE EDGE FORWARD.

The first attempt of the beginner is to walk, and this walk shortly becomes a sliding gait, done entirely on the inside edge of the skate.

The first impulse is to be gained by pressing the inside edge of one skate against the ice, and advancing with the opposite foot. To effect this, the beginner must bring the feet nearly together, turn the left somewhat out, place the right a little in advance and at right angles with it, lean forward with the right shoulder, and at the same time move the right foot onwards, and press sharply, or strike the ice with the inside edge of the left skate,—care being taken instantly to throw the weight on the right foot. (Plate XIX. fig. 1.) While thus in motion, the skater must bring up the left foot nearly to a level with the other, and may for the present proceed a short way on both feet.

He must next place the left foot in advance in its turn, bring the left shoulder forward, inclining to that side, strike from the inside edge of the right skate, and proceed as before.

Finally, this motion has only to be repeated on each foot alternately, gradually keeping the foot from which he

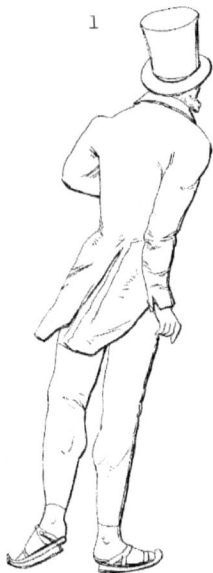

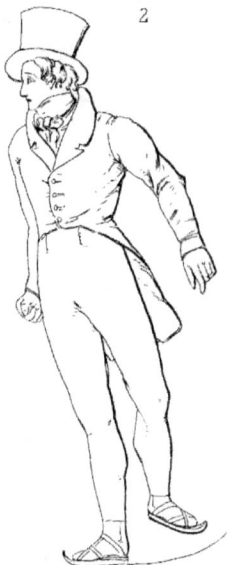

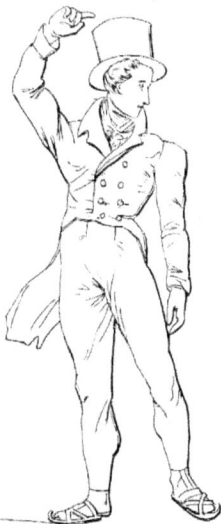

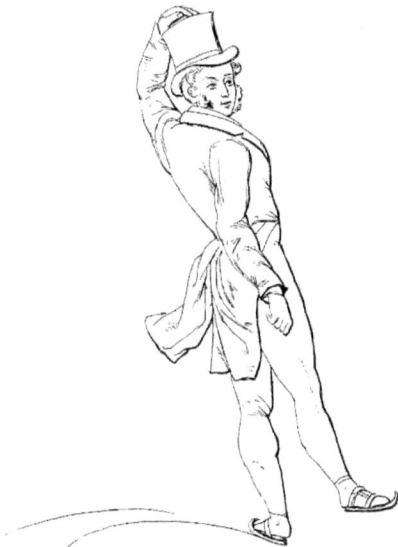

struck longer off the ice, till he has gained sufficient command of himself to keep it off altogether, and is able to strike directly from one to the other, without at any time having them both on the ice together. Having practiced this till he has gained some degree of firmness and power, and a command of his balance, he may proceed to

THE FORWARD ROLL, OR OUTSIDE EDGE.

This is commonly reckoned the first step to figure skating, as, when it is once effected, the rest follows with ease. The impulse is gained in the same manner as for the ordinary run; but, to get on the outside edge of the right foot, the moment that foot is in motion, the skater must advance the left shoulder, throw the right·arm back, look over the right shoulder, and incline the whole person boldly and decisively on that side, keeping the left foot suspended behind. (Plate XIX. fig. 2.)

As he proceeds, he must bring the left foot past the inside of the right, with a slight jerk, which produces an opposing balance of the body; the right foot must quickly press, first on the outside of the heel, then on the inside, or its toe; the left foot must be placed down in front, before it is removed more than about eight or ten inches from the other foot; and, by striking outside to the left, giving at the same moment a strong push with the inside of the right toe, the skater passes from right to left, inclining to the left side, in the same manner as he did to the right. He then continues to change from left to right, and from right to left, in the same manner. At first he should not remain long upon one leg, nor scruple occasionally to put the other down to assist; and throughout he must keep himself erect, leaning most on the heel.

The Dutch travelling roll is done on the outside edge

9

forward, in a manner just represented, except that there is
described a small segment of a very large circle, thus:

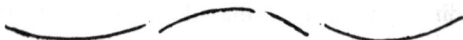

diverging from the straight line no more than is requisite
to keep the skate on its edge.

The cross roll on figure 8 is also done on the outside edge
forward.   This is only the completion of the circle on the
outside edge; and it is performed by crossing the legs, and
striking from the outside instead of the inside edge.   In
order to do this, as the skater draws to the close of the
stroke on his right leg, he must throw the left quite across
it, which will cause him to press hard on the outside of the
right skate, from which he must immediately strike, at the
same time throwing back the left arm, and looking over the
left shoulder, to bring him well upon the outside of that
skate.   By completing the circle in this manner on each
leg, the 8 is formed:

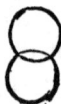

each circle being small, complete, and well-formed, before
the foot is changed.

The Mercury figure is merely the outside and inside forward succeeding each other on the same leg alternately, by
which a serpentine line is described, thus:

Outside.   *Inside.*   *Outside.*

This is skated with the force and rapidity gained by a
run.   When the run is complete, and the skater on the

outside edge, his person becomes quiescent, in the attitude
of Mercury, having the right arm advanced and much
raised, the face turned over the right shoulder, and the left
foot off the ice, a short distance behind the other, turned
out and pointed.

FIGURE OF THREE, OR INSIDE EDGE BACKWARDS.

This figure is formed by turning from the outside edge
forward to the inside edge backward on the same foot. The
head of the 3 is formed like the half circle, on the heel of
the outside edge; but when the half circle is complete, the
skater leans suddenly forward, and rests on the same toe
inside, and a backward motion, making the tail of the 3, is
the consequence. The figure described by the right leg
should be nearly in the form of No. 1; and on the left leg
should be reversed, and resemble No. 2.

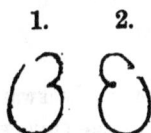

1.   2.

At first, the skater should not throw himself quite so hard
as hitherto on the outside forward, in order that he may
be able the more easily to change to the inside back. He
may also be for some time contented with much less than
a semi-circle before he turns. Having done this, and
brought the left leg nearly up to the other, he must not
pass it on in advance, as he would to complete a circle, but
throw it gently off sidewise, at the same moment turning
the face from the right to the left shoulder, and giving the
whole person a slight inclination to the left side. These
motions throw the skater upon the inside of his skate;

but as the first impulse should still retain most of its force, he continues to move on the inside back, in a direction so little different, that his first impulse loses little by the change. (Plate XIX. fig. 1.)

If unable to change the edge by this method, the skater may assist himself by slightly and gently swinging the arm and leg outward, so as to incline the person to a rotary motion. This swing, however, must be corrected as soon as the object is attained; and it must generally be observed that the change from edge to edge is to be effected merely by the inclination of the body, not by swinging.

When the skater is able to join the ends of the 3, so as to form one side of a circle, then, by striking off in the same manner, and completing another 3, with the left leg, the combination of the two 3's will form an 8. In the first attempts, the 3 should not be made above two feet long, which he will acquire the power of doing almost imperceptibly. He may then gradually extend the size as he advances in the art.

Though, in this section, backward skating is spoken of, the term refers to the skate only, which in such case moves heel foremost, but the person of the skater moves sidewise, the face being always turned in the direction in which he is proceeding.

OUTSIDE EDGE BACKWARDS.

Here the skater, having completed the 3, and being carried on by the first impulse, still continues his progress in the same direction, but on the other foot, putting it down on its outside edge, and continuing to go backwards slowly.

To accomplish this, the skater, after making the 3, and placing the outside edge of his left foot on the ice, should at once turn his face over the right shoulder, raise his right foot from the ice, and throw back his right arm and shoulder. (Plate XIX. fig. 2.) If, for awhile, he is unable readily to raise that foot which has made the 3, and leave himself on the outside of the other skate, he may keep both down for some distance, putting himself, however, in attitude of being on the outside only of one skate, and gradually lifting the other off the ice as he acquires ability.

When finishing any figure, this use of both feet backward has great convenience and beauty.

Before venturing on the outside backward, the skater, ought to take care that the ice is clear of stones, reeds, &c. and also be certain of the good quality of his irons. When going with great force backward, the course may be deflected, so as to stop by degrees; and, when moving slowly, the suspended foot may be put down in a cross direction to the path.

Such are the four movements of which alone the skate is capable: namely, the inside edge forward; the outside forward; the inside back; and the outside back; in which has been seen how the impulse for the first two is gained, and how the third flows from the second, and the fourth from the third. By the combination of these elements of skating, and the variations with which they succeed each other, are formed all the evolutions in this art.

The Double Three is that combination in which the skates are brought from the inside back of the first three, to the outside forward of the second. Here the skater, after having completed one 3, and being on the inside back, must bring the whole of the left side forward, particularly the leg, till it is thrown almost across the right, on which he is skating. This action brings him once more to the outside forward, from which he again turns to the inside back. While he is still in motion on the second inside

9*

back of the right leg, he must strike on the left, and repeat the same on that.

It is at first enough to do two 3's perfectly and smoothly. Their number from one impulse may be increased as the skater gains steadiness and skill; the art of accomplishing this being to touch as lightly as possible on each side of the skate successively, so that the first impulse may be preserved and made the most of.

The Back Roll is a means of moving from one foot to another.

Suppose the skater to have put himself on the outside edge back of the left leg, with considerable impulse, by means of the 3 performed on the right,—not bearing hard on the edge, for the object is to change it, and take up the motion on the right foot,—this is effected by throwing the left arm and shoulder back, and turning the face to look over them; when, having brought the inside of his left skate to bear on the ice, he must immediately strike from it to the outside back of the other, by pressing it into the ice as forcibly as he can at the toe. Having thus been brought to the backward roll on the right foot, he repeats the same with it.

The Back Cross Roll is done by changing the balance of the body, to move from one foot to the other, in the same manner as for the back roll. The stroke is from the outside instead of the inside edge of the skate; the edge on which he is skating not being changed, but the right foot, which is off the ice, being crossed at the back of the left, and put down, and the stroke taken at the same moment, from the outside edge of the left skate, at the toe. As in the back roll of both forms, the strokes are but feeble, the skater may, from time to time, renew his impulse as he finds occasion, by commencing anew with the 3.

The large outside backward roll is attained by a run, when the skater, having gained all the impulse he can, strikes on the outside forward of the right leg, turns the 3, and immediately puts down the left on the outside back. He then, without further effort, flies rapidly over the ice; the left arm being raised, the head turned over the right shoulder, and the right foot turned out and pointed.

It must be evident, that the elements described may be combined and varied infinitely. Hence waltz and quadrille skating, &c., which may be described as combinations of 8's, outside backwards, &c. These are left to the judgment of the skater, and his skill in the art.

In the North it is common to travel in skates on the gulfs and rivers; and, with a favorable wind, they go faster than vessels. It is a kind of flight, for they only touch the ground in a very slight thin line. As to feats in skating, we are told, that the Frieslander, who is generally a skillful skater, often goes for a long time at the rate of fifteen miles an hour. In 1801, two young women, going thirty miles in two hours, won the prize in a skating race at Groningen. In 1821, a Lincolnshire man, for a wager of 100 guineas, skated one mile within two seconds of three minutes.

DANGERS IN SKATING.

If the chest be irritable, it is neither salutary nor easy to skate against the wind. In countries where these exercises are general, inflammations of the chest are very common in winter. Skating sometimes exposes to much danger. If the skater find that he cannot get away from rotten ice, he must crawl over it on his hands and knees, in order to reduce his weight on the supporting points. If he fall on it at length, he must roll away from it towards ice more firm. If he fall into a hole, he must extend his arms horizontally over the edges of the unbroken ice, and only tread water till a ladder or a plank is pushed towards him, or a rope is thrown for his hold.

TREATMENT RECOMMENDED IN THE CASE OF DROWNED PERSONS.

CAUTIONS.—1. Lose no time. 2. Avoid all rough usage. 3. Never hold the body up by the feet. 4. Never roll the body on casks. 5. Nor rub the body with salt or spirits. 6. Nor inject tobacco-smoke or infusion of tobacco.

RESTORATIVE MEANS IF APPARENTLY DROWNED.—Send quickly for medical assistance; but do not delay the following means.

I. Convey the body carefully, with the head and shoulders supported in a raised position, to the nearest house.

II. Strip the body, and rub it dry; then wrap it in hot blankets and place it in a warm bed in a warm chamber.

III. Wipe and cleanse the mouth and nostrils.

IV. In order to restore the natural warmth of the body:

1. Move a heated covered warming-pan over the back and spine.

2. Put bladders or bottles of hot water, or heated bricks, to the pit of the stomach, the arm-pits, between the thighs, and to the soles of the feet.

3. Foment the body with hot flannels; but, if possible,

4. Immerse the body in a warm bath, as hot as the hand can bear without pain, as this is preferable to the other means for restoring warmth.

5. Rub the body briskly with the hand; do not, however, suspend the use of the other means at the same time.

V. In order to restore breathing, introduce the pipe of a common bellows (where the apparatus of the Society is not at hand) into one nostril, carefully closing the other and the mouth: at the same time draw downwards and push gently backwards the upper part of the windpipe, to allow a more free admission of air: blow the bellows gently in order to inflate the lungs, till the breast be a little raised: the mouth and nostrils should then be set free, and a moderate pressure should be made with the hand upon the chest. Repeat this process till life appears.

VI. Electricity should be employed early by a medical assistant.

VII. Inject into the stomach, by means of an elastic tube and syringe, half a pint of warm brandy and water, or wine and water.

VIII. Apply sal-volatile or hartshorn to the nostrils.

IF APPARENTLY DEAD FROM INTENSE COLD.—Rub the body with snow, ice, or cold water. Restore warmth by slow degrees; and after some time, if necessary, employ the means recommended for the drowned. In these accidents, it is highly dangerous to apply heat too early.

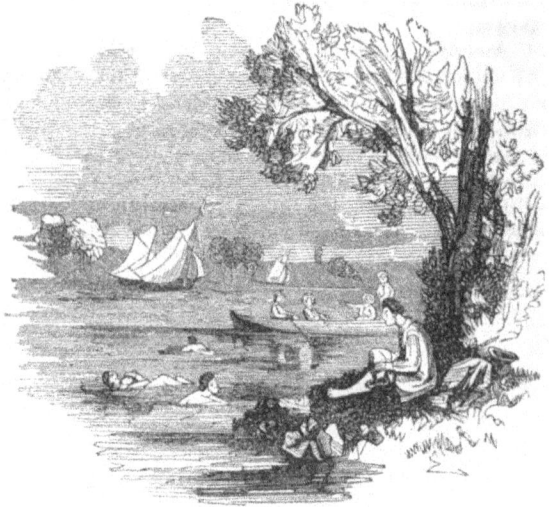

SWIMMING.

SWIMMING, considered with regard to the movements that it requires, is useful in promoting great muscular strength; but the good effects are not solely the result of the exercise that the muscles receive, but partly of the medium in which the body is moved. But the considerable increase of general force, and the tranquilizing of the nervous system produced by swimming, arise chiefly from this, that the movements, in consequence of the cold and dense medium in which they take place, occasion no loss.* It is easy to conceive of what utility swimming must be, where the very high state of the atmospheric temperature requires

---

* The expression "loss" here, is used as the result produced by increased evaporation from the pores, consequent upon violent bodily exertion.

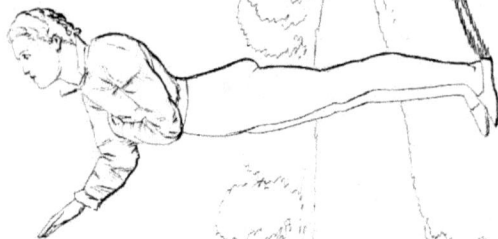

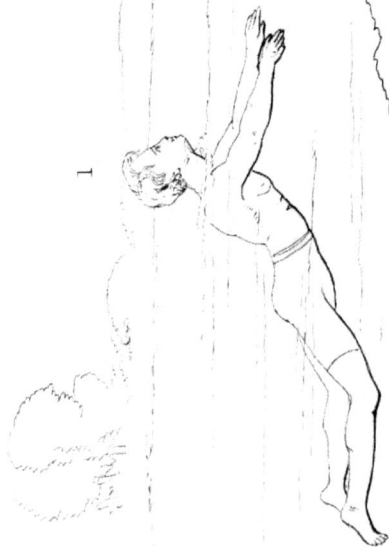

inactivity in consequence of the excessive loss caused by the slightest movement. It then becomes an exceedingly valuable resource, the only one, indeed, by which muscular weakness can be remedied, and the energy of the vital functions maintained. We must therefore regard swimming as one of the most beneficial exercises that can be taken in summer.

The ancients, particularly the Athenians, regarded swimming as indispensable; and when they wished to designate a man who was fit for nothing, they used to say, " he cannot even swim," or "he can neither read nor swim." At many seaports, the art of swimming is almost indispensable; and the sailors' children are as familiar with the water as with the air. Copenhagen is perhaps the only place where sailors are trained by rules of art; and there, this exercise is more general and in greater perfection than elsewhere. It may here be observed, that it is not fear alone that prevents a man swimming. Swimming is an art that must be learnt; and fear is only an obstacle to the learning.

PREPARATORY INSTRUCTIONS AS TO ATTITUDE AND ACTION IN SWIMMING.

As it is on the movements of the limbs, and a certain attitude of the body, that the power of swimming depends, its first principles may evidently be acquired out of the water.

Attitude.

The head must be drawn back, and the chin elevated, the breast projected, and the back hollowed and kept steady. (Plate XX. figs. 1 and 2.) The head can scarcely be thrown too much back, or the back too much hollowed. Those who do otherwise, swim with their feet near the surface of the water, instead of having them too or three feet deep.

Action of the Hands.

In the proper position of the hands, the fingers must be kept close, with the thumbs by the edge of the fore-fingers; and the hands made concave on their inside, though not so much as to diminish their size and power in swimming. The hands, thus formed, should be placed just before the breast, the wrist touching it, and the fingers pointing forward. (Plate XXI. fig. 1.)

The first elevation is formed by raising the ends of the fingers three or four inches higher than the rest of the hands. The second, by raising the outer edge of the hand two or three inches higher than the inner edge.

The formation of the hands, their first position, and their two modes of elevation, being clearly understood, the forward stroke is next made, by projecting them in that direction to their utmost extent, employing therein their first elevation, in order to produce buoyancy, but taking care the fingers do not break the surface of the water. (Plate XXI. fig. 2.) In the outward stroke of the hands, the second elevation must be employed; and, in it, they must sweep downward and outward as low as, but at a distance from the hips, both laterally and anteriorly. (Plate XXI. figs. 3 and 4.)

The retraction of the hands is effected by bringing the arms closer to the sides, bending the elbow joints upwards and the wrists downwards, so that the hands hang down, while the arms are raising them to the first position, the action of the hands being gentle and easy. In the three

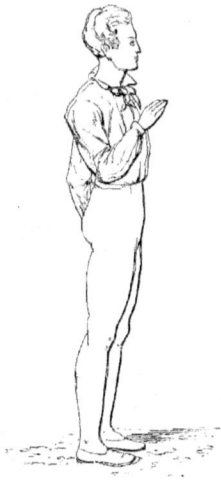

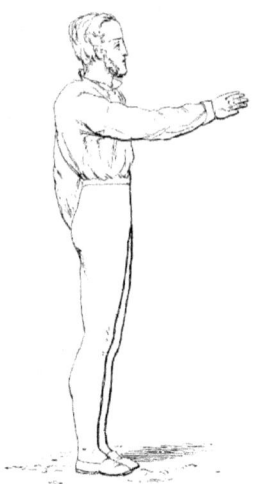

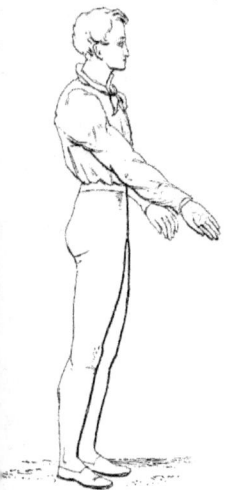

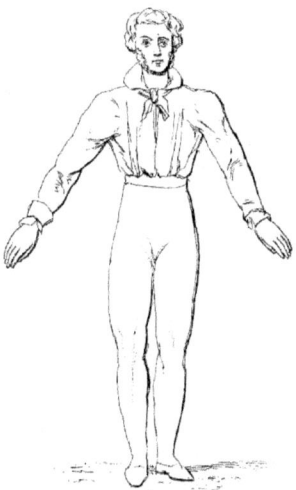

movements just described, one arm may be exercised at a time, until each is accustomed to the action.

Action of the Feet.

In drawing up the legs, the knees must be inclined inward, and the soles of the feet outward. (Plate XXII. fig. 1.) The throwing out the feet should be to the extent of the legs, as widely from each other as possible. (Plate XXII. fig. 2.) The bringing down the legs must be done briskly, until they come close together. In drawing up the legs, there is a loss of power; in throwing out the legs, there is a gain equal to that loss; and in bringing down the legs, there is an evident gain.

The arms and legs should act alternately; the arms descending while the legs are rising—(Plate XXII. fig. 3;) and, oppositely, the arms rising while the legs are descending. (Plate XXII. fig. 4.) Thus the action of both is unceasingly interchanged; and, until great facility in this interchange is effected, no one can swim smoothly, or keep the body in one continued progressive motion. In practising the action of the legs, one hand may rest on the top of a chair, while the opposite leg is exercised. When both the arms and the legs are separately accustomed to the action, the arm and leg of the same side may be exercised together.

PLACE AND TIME OF SWIMMING.

Place.

Of all places for swimming, the sea is the best; running waters next; and ponds the worst. In these a particular spot should be chosen, where there is not much stream, and which is known to be safe.

The swimmer should make sure that the bottom is not

out of his depth; and, on this subject, he cannot be too
cautious when he has no one with him who knows the
place. If capable of diving, he should ascertain if the
water be sufficiently deep for that purpose, otherwise, he
may injure himself against the bottom. The bottom should
be of gravel, or smooth stones, and free from holes, so that
he may be in no danger of sinking in the mud or wounding
the feet. Of weeds he must beware; for if his feet get
entangled among them, no aid, even if near, may be able
to extricate him.

Time.

The best season of the year for swimming is during the
months of May, June, July, and August. Morning before
breakfast—that is to say, from seven till eight o'clock—is
the time. In the evening, the hair is not perfectly dried,
and coryza is sometimes the consequence. Bathing during
rain is bad, for it chills the water, and, by wetting the
clothes, endangers catching cold. In practising swimming
during those hours of the day when the heat of the sun is
felt most sensibly, if the hair be thick, it should be kept
constantly wet; if the head be bald, it must be covered
with a handkerchief, and frequently wetted.

It is advisable not to enter the water before digestion is
finished. The danger is this case arises less from the violent movements which generally disorder digestion, than
from the impression produced by the medium in which
these movements are executed. It is not less so when very
hot, or quite cold. It is wrong to enter the water in a
perspiration, however trifling it may be. After violent
exercises, it is better to wash and employ friction than to
bathe. Persons of plethoric temperament, who are subject
to periodical evacuations, such as hemorrhoids, or even to

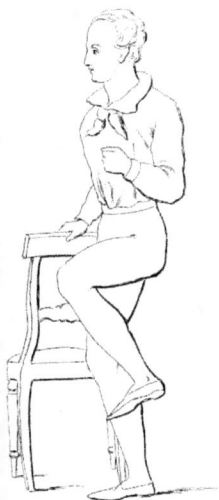

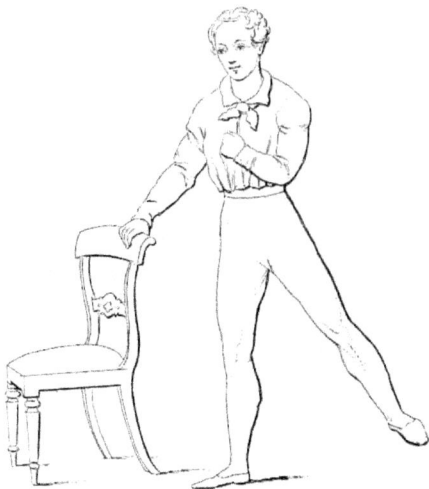

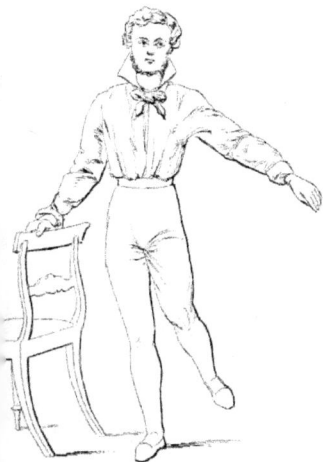

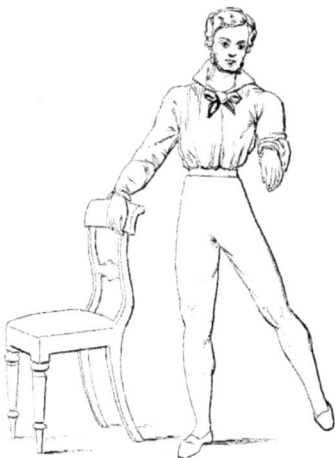

cutaneous eruptions, will do well to abstain from swimming during the appearance of these affections.

Dress.

Every swimmer should use short drawers, and might, in particular places, use canvass slippers. It is even of great importance to be able to swim in jacket and trousers.

Aids.

The aid of the hand is much preferable to corks or bladders, because it can be withdrawn gradually and insensibly. With this view, a grown-up person may take the learner in his arms, carry him into the water breast high, place him nearly flat upon it, support him by one hand under the breast, and direct him as to attitude and action. If the support of the hand be very gradually withdrawn, the swimmer will, in the course of the first ten days, find it quite unnecessary. When the aid of the hand cannot be obtained, inflated membranes or corks may be employed. The only argument for their use is, that attitude and action may be perfected while the body is thus supported; and that, with some contrivance, they also may gradually be laid aside, though by no means so easily as the hand.

The best mode of employing corks is to choose a piece about a foot long, and six or seven inches broad; to fasten a band across the middle of it; to place it on the back, so that the upper end may come between the shoulder-blades, where the edge may be rounded; and to tie the band over the breast. Over this, several other pieces of cork, each smaller than the preceding, may be fixed, so that, as the swimmer improves, he may leave them off one by one. Even with all these aids, the young swimmer should never venture out of his depth, if he cannot swim without them.

Cramp.

As to cramp, those chiefly are liable to it who plunge into the water when they are heated, who remain in it till they are benumbed with cold, or who exhaust themselves by violent exercise. Persons subject to this affection must be careful with regard to the selection of the place where they bathe, if they are not sufficiently skillful in swimming to vary their attitudes, and dispense instantly with the use of the limb attacked by cramp. Even when this does occur, the skillful swimmer knows how to reach the shore by the aid of the limbs which are unaffected, while the uninstructed one is liable to be drowned.

If attacked in this way in the leg, the swimmer must strike out the limb with all his strength, thrusting the heel downward and drawing the toes upward, notwithstanding the momentary pain it may occasion; or he may immediately turn flat on his back, and jerk out the affected limb in the air, taking care not to elevate it so high as greatly to disturb the balance of the body. If this does not succeed, he must paddle ashore with his hands, or keep himself afloat by their aid, until assistance can reach him. Should he even be unable to float on his back, he must put himself in the upright position, and keep his head above the surface by merely striking the water downward with his hands at the hips, without any assistance from the legs.

PROCEDURE WHEN IN THE WATER, AND USUAL MODE OF FRONT SWIMMING.

Entering the Water.

Instructors should never force young swimmers reluctantly to leap into the water. It would be advisable for delicate persons, especially when they intend to plunge in, to put a little cotton steeped in oil, and afterwards pressed, in their ears, before entering the water. This precaution will prevent irritation of the organ of hearing. In entering, the head should be wetted first, either by plunging in head foremost, or by pouring water on it, in order to prevent the pressure of the water driving up the blood into it too quickly, and increasing congestion. The swimmer should next advance, by a clear shelving shore or bank, where he has ascertained the depth by plumbing or otherwise, till the water reaches his breast; should turn towards the place of entrance; and, having inflated his breast, lay it upon the water, suffering that to rise to his chin, the lips being closed.

Buoyancy in the Water.

The head alone is specifically heavier than salt water. Even the legs and arms are specifically lighter; and the trunk is still more so. Thus the body cannot sink in salt water, even if the lungs were filled, except owing to the excessive specific gravity of the head.

Not only the head, but the legs and arms, are specifically heavier than fresh water; but still the hollowness of the trunk renders the body altogether too light to sink wholly under water, so that some part remains above until the lungs become filled. In general, when the human body is immersed, one-eleventh of its weight remains above the surface in fresh water, and one-tenth in salt water.

In salt water, therefore, a person throwing himself on his back, and extending his arms, may easily lie so as to keep his mouth and nostrils free from breathing; and, by a small motion of the hand, may prevent turning, if he perceive any tendency to it. In fresh water, a man cannot

10*

long continue in that situation, except by the action of his hands; and if no such action be employed, the legs and lower part of the body will gradually sink into an upright position, the hollow of the breast keeping the head uppermost. If, however, in this position, the head be kept upright above the shoulders, as in standing on the ground, the immersion, owing to the weight of the part of the head out of the water, will reach above the mouth and nostrils, perhaps a little above the eyes. On the contrary, in the same position, if the head be leaned back, so that the face is turned upwards, the back part of the head has its weight supported by the water, and the face will rise an inch higher at every inspiration, and will sink as much at every expiration, but never so low that the water can come over the mouth.

For all these reasons, though the impetus given by the fall of the body into water occasions its sinking to a depth proportioned to the force of the descent, its natural buoyancy soon impels it again to the surface, where, after a few oscillations up and down, it settles with the head free.

Unfortunately, ignorant people stretch the arms out to grasp at anything or nothing, and thereby keep the head under; for the arms and head, together exceeding in weight one-tenth of the body, cannot remain above the surface at the same time. The buoyancy of the trunk, then and then only, occasions the head and shoulders to sink, the ridge of the bent back becoming the portion exposed; and, in this attitude, water is swallowed, by which the specifie gravity is increased, and the body settles to the bottom. It is, therefore, most important to the safety of the inexperienced to be firmly convinced that the body naturally floats.

To satisfy the beginner of the truth of this, Dr. Franklin

advises him to choose a place where clear water deepens gradually, to walk into it till it is up to his breast, to turn his face to the shore, and to throw an egg into the water between him and it—so deep that he cannot fetch it up by diving. To encourage him to take it up, he must reflect that his progress will be from deep to shallow water, and that at any time he may, by bringing his legs under him, and standing on the bottom, raise his head far above the water. He must then plunge under it, having his eyes open, before as well as after going under; throw himself towards the egg, and endeavor, by the action of his hands and feet against the water, to get forward till within reach of it. In this attempt, he will find that the water brings him up against his inclination, that it is not so easy to sink as he imagined, and that he cannot, but by force, get down to the egg. Thus he feels the power of water to support him, and learns to confide in that power; while his endeavors to overcome it, and reach the egg, teach him the manner of acting on the water with his feet and hands, as he afterwards must in swimming, in order to support his head higher above the water, or to go forward through it.

If then, any person, however unacquainted with swimming, will hold himself perfectly still and upright, as if standing with his head somewhat thrown back so as to rest on the surface, his face will remain above the water, and he will enjoy full freedom of breathing. To do this most effectually, the head must be so far thrown back that the chin is higher than the forehead, the breast inflated, the back quite hollow, and the hands and arms kept under water. If these directions be carefully observed, the face will float above the water, and the body will settle in a diagonal direction. (Plate XXIII. fig. 1.)

In this case, the only difficulty is to preserve the balance

of the body. This is secured, as described by Bernardi,
by extending the arms laterally under the surface of the
water, with the legs separated, the one to the front and the
other behind : thus presenting resistance to any tendency
of the body to incline to either side, forward or backward.
This posture may be preserved any length of time. (Plate
XXIII. fig. 2.)

The Abbé Paul Moccia, who lived in Naples in 1760,
perceived, at the age of fifty, that he could never entirely
cover himself in the water. He weighed three hundred
pounds (Italian weight,) but being very fat, he lost at least
thirty pounds in the water. Robertson had just made his
experiments on the specific weight of man; and everybody
was then occupied with the Abbé, who could walk in the
water with nearly half his body out of it.

Attitude and Action in the Water.

The swimmer having, by all the preceding means,
acquired confidence, may now practice the instructions
already given on attitude and action in swimming : or he
may first proceed with the system of Bernardi, which immediately follows. As the former have already been given
in ample detail, there is nothing new here to be added respecting them, except that, while the attitude is correct,
the limbs must be exercised calmly, and free from all hurry
and trepidation, the breath being held, and the breast kept
inflated, while a few strokes are made. In swimming in
the usual way, there is, first, extension, flexion, abduction
and adduction of the members; secondly, almost constant
dilation of the chest, to diminish the mobility of the point
of attachment of the muscles which are inserted in the
elastic sides of this cavity, and to render the body specifically lighter; thirdly, constant action of the muscles of

the back part of the neck, to raise the head, which is relatively very heavy, and to allow the air free entrance to the lungs.

Respiration in Swimming.

If the breath is drawn at the moment when the swimmer strikes out with the legs, instead of when the body is elevated by the hands descending towards the hips, the head partially sinks, the face is driven against the water, and the mouth becomes filled. If, on the contrary, the breath is drawn when the body is elevated by the hands descending towards the hips, when the progress of the body forward consequently ceases, when the face is no longer driven against the water, but is elevated above the surface,—then, not only cannot the water enter, but if the mouth were at other times even with, or partly under the surface, no water could enter it, as the air, at such times, driven outward between the lips, would effectually prevent it. The breath should accordingly be expired while the body, at the next stroke, is sent forward by the action of the legs.

Coming out of the Water.

Too much fatigue in the water weakens the strength and presence of mind necessary to avoid accidents. A person who is fatigued, and remains there without motion, soon becomes weak and chilly. As soon as he feels fatigued, chill, or numb, he should quit the water, and dry and dress himself as quickly as possible. Friction, previous to dressing, drives the blood over every part of the body, creates an agreeable glow, and strengthens the joints and muscles.

UPRIGHT SWIMMING.

Bernardi's System.

The principal reasons given by Bernardi for recommending the upright position in swimming are—its conformity to the accustomed movement of the limbs; the freedom it gives to the hands and arms, by which any impediment may be moved, or any offered aid readily laid hold of; vision all round; a much greater facility of breathing; and lastly, that much less of the body is exposed to the risk of being laid hold of by persons struggling in the water.

The less we alter our method of advancing in the water from what is habitual to us on shore, the more easy do we find a continued exercise of it. The most important consequence of this is, that, though a person swimming in an upright posture advances more slowly, he is able to continue his course much longer ; and certainly nothing can be more beneficial to a swimmer than whatever tends to husband his strength, and to enable him to remain long in the water with safety.

Bernardi's primary object is to enable the pupil to float in an upright posture, and to feel confidence in the buoyancy of his body. He accordingly supports the pupil under the shoulders until he floats tranquilly with the head and part of the neck above the surface, the arms being stretched out horizontally under water. From time to time, the supporting arm is removed, but again restored, so as never to suffer the head to sink, which would disturb the growing confidence, and give rise to efforts destructive of the success of the lesson. In this early stage, the unsteadiness of the body is the chief difficulty to be overcome.

The head is the great regulator of our movements in water. Its smallest inclination to either side instantly operates on the whole body; and, if not corrected, throws it into a horizontal posture. The pupil must, therefore, restore any disturbance of equilibrium, by a cautious movement of the head alone in an opposite direction. This first lesson being familiarized by practice, he is taught the use of the legs and arms for balancing the body in the water. One leg being stretched forward, the other backward, and the arms laterally, he soon finds himself steadily sustained, and independent of further aid in floating.

When these first steps have been gained, the sweeping semi-circular motion of the arms is shown. This is practised slowly, without motion forwards, until attained with precision. After this, a slight inclination of the body from the upright position occasions its advancing. The motion of striking with the legs is added in the same measured manner; so that the pupil is not perplexed by the acquisition of more than one thing at a time. In this method, the motions of both arms and legs differ from those we have so carefully described, only in so far as they are modified by a more upright position. It is optional, therefore, with the reader, to practise either method. The general principles of both are now before him.

The upright position a little inclined backwards, (which, like every other change of posture, must be done deliberately, by the corresponding movement of the head,) reversing in this case the motion of the arms, and striking the flat part of the foot down and a little forward, gives the motion backward, which is performed with greater ease than when the body is laid horizontally on the back. According to this system, Bernardi says, a swimmer ought at every stroke to urge himself forward a distance equal to the length of his body. A good swimmer ought to make about three miles an hour. A good day's journey may thus be achieved, if the strength be used with due discretion, and the swimmer be familiar with the various means by which it may be recruited.

Of Bernardi's successful practice, he says, " Having been appointed to instruct the youths of the Royal Naval Academy of Naples in the art of swimming, a trial of the proficiency of the pupils took place, under the inspection of a number of people assembled on the shore for that purpose, on the tenth day of their instruction. A twelve-oared boat attended the progress of the pupils, from motives of precaution. They swam so far out in the bay, that at length the heads of the young men could with difficulty be discerned with the naked eye; and the Major-General of Marine, Forteguerri, for whose inspection the exhibition was intended, expressed serious apprehensions for their safety. Upon their return to the shore, the young men, however, assured him that they felt so little exhausted as to be willing immediately to repeat the exertion." An official report on the subject has also been drawn up by commission (appointed by the Neapolitan government,) after devoting a month to the investigation of Bernardi's plan; and it states as follows:

" 1st. It has been established by the experience of more than a hundred persons of different bodily constitutions, that the human body is lighter than water, and consequently will float by nature; but that the art of swimming must be acquired, to render that privilege useful.

" 2dly. That Bernardi's system is new, in so far as it is founded on the principle of husbanding the strength, and rendering the power of recruiting it easy. The speed, according to the new method, is no doubt diminished; but

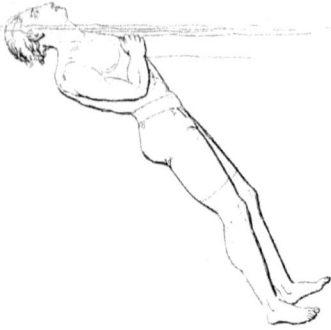

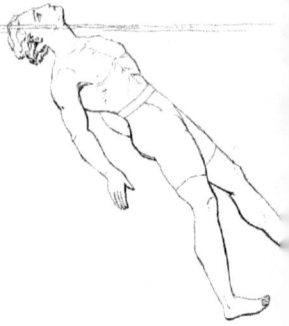

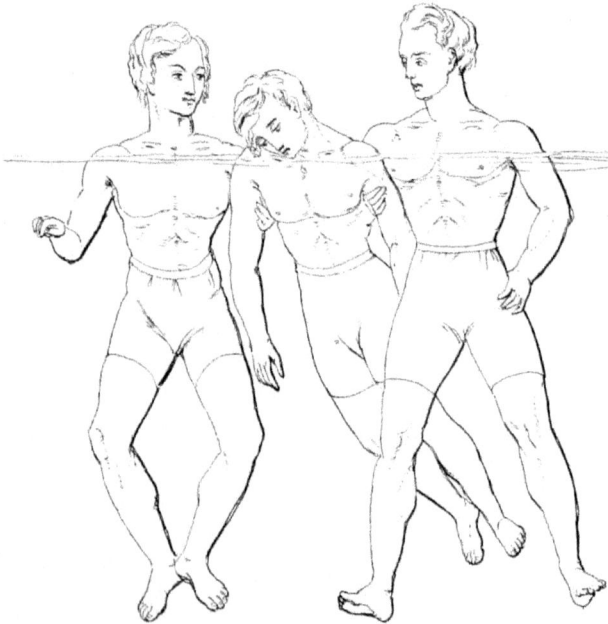

security is much more important than speed; and the new plan is not exclusive of the old, when occasions require great effort.

"3dly. That the new method is sooner learnt than the old, to the extent of advancing a pupil in one day as far as a month's instruction on the old plan."

Treading Water.

This differs little from the system just described. As in it, the position is upright; but progression is obtained by the action of the legs alone. There is little power in this method of swimming: but it may be very useful in rescuing drowning persons.

The arms should be folded across, below the breast, or compressed against the hips, and the legs employed as in front swimming, except as to time and extent. They should perform their action in half the usual time, or two strokes should be taken in the time of one; because, acting perpendicularly, each stroke would otherwise raise the swimmer too much, and he would sink too low between the strokes, were they not quickly to follow each other. They should also work in about two-thirds of the usual space, preserving the upper or stronger, and omitting the lower or weaker part of the stroke.

There is, however, another mode of treading water, in which the thighs are separated, and the legs slightly bent, or curved together, as in a half-sitting posture. Here the legs are used alternately, so that, while one remains more contracted, the other, less so, describes a circle. By this method the swimmer does not seem to hop in the water, but remains nearly at the same height. Pl. XXIII. fig. 3, represents both these methods, and shows their peculiar adaptation to relieve drowning persons.

11

BACK SWIMMING.

In swimming on the back, the action of the thoracic member is weaker, because the swimmer can support himself on the water without their assistance. The muscular contractions take place principally in the muscles of the abdominal members, and in those of the anterior part of the neck. Though little calculated for progression, it is the easiest of all methods, because, much of the head being immersed, little effort is required for support. For this purpose, the swimmer must lie down gently upon the water; the body extended; the head kept in a line with it, so that the back and much of the upper part of the head may be immersed; the head and breast must remain perfectly unagitated by the action of the legs; the hand laid on the thighs, (Plate XXIV. fig. 1,) and the legs employed as in front swimming, care being taken that the knees do not rise out of the water. (Plate XXIV. fig. 2.) The arms may, however, be used in various ways in swimming on the back.

In the method called winging, the arms are extended till in a line with each other; they must then be struck down to the thighs, with the palms turned in that direction, and the thumbs inclining downward to increase the buoyancy, (Plate XXIV. fig. 3;) the palms must then be moved edgewise, and the arms elevated as before, (Plate XXIV. fig. 4,) and so on, repeating the same actions. The legs should throughout make one stroke as the arms are struck down, and another as they are elevated. The other mode, called finning, differs from this only in the stroke of the arms being shorter, and made in the same time as that of the legs.

In back swimming, the body should be extended after each stroke, and long pauses made between these. The act of passing from front to back, or back to front swimming,

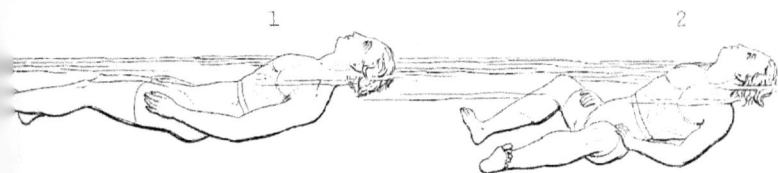

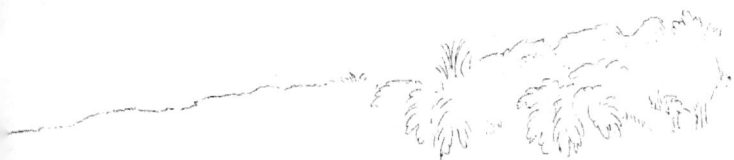

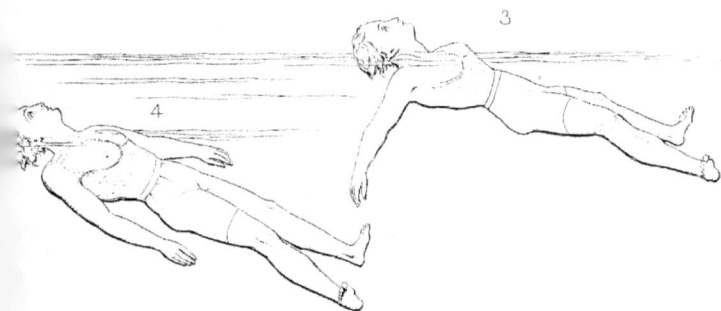

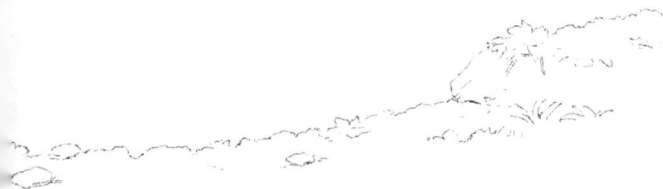

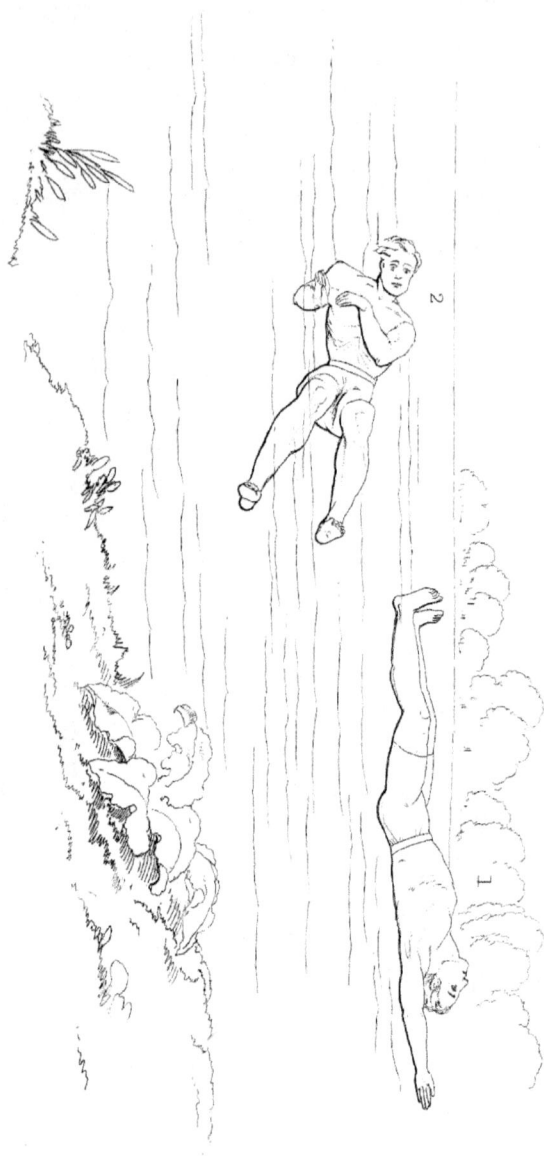

must always be performed immediately after throwing out the feet. To turn from the breast to the back, the legs must be raised forward, and the head thrown backward, until the body is in a right position. To turn from the back to the breast, the legs must be dropped, and the body thrown forward on the breast.

FLOATING.

Floating is properly a transition from swimming on the back. To effect it, it is necessary, while the legs are gently exercising, to extend the arms as far as possible beyond the head, equi-distant from, and parallel with its sides, but never rising above the surface; to immerse the head rather deeply, and elevate the chin more than the forehead; to inflate the chest while taking this position, and so to keep it as much as possible; and to cease the action of the legs, and put the feet together. (Plate XXV. fig. 1.) The swimmer will thus be able to float, rising a little with every inspiration, and falling with every expiration. Should the feet descend, the loins may be hollowed.

SIDE SWIMMING.

For this purpose, the body may be turned either upon the right or left side: the feet must perform their usual motions: the arms also require peculiar guidance. In lowering the left, and elevating the right side, the swimmer must strike forward with the left hand, and sideways with the right; the back of the latter being front, instead of upward, and the thumb side of the hand downward to serve as an oar. In turning on the right side, the swimmer must strike out with the right hand, and use the left as an oar. In both cases, the lower arm stretches itself out quickly, at the same time that the feet are striking; and the upper arm strikes at the same time that the feet are impelling, the hand of the latter arm beginning its stroke on a level with the head.   While this hand is again brought forward, and the feet are contracted, the lower hand is drawn back towards the breast, rather to sustain than to impel. (Plate XXV. fig. 2.)   As side swimming presents to the water a smaller surface than front swimming, it is preferable when rapidity is necessary.   But, though generally adopted when it is required to pass over a short distance with rapidity, it is much more fatiguing than the preceding methods.

PLUNGING.

In the leap to plunge the legs must be kept together, the arms close, and the plunge made either with the feet or the head foremost.   With the feet foremost they must be kept together, and the body inclined backwards.   With the head foremost, the methods vary.

In the deep plunge, which is used where it is known that there is depth of water, the swimmer has his arms outstretched, his knees bent, and his body lent forwards, (Plate XXVI. fig. 1,) till the head descends nearly to the feet, when the spine and knees are extended.   This plunge may be made without the slightest noise.   When the swimmer rises to the surface, he must not open his mouth before previously repelling the water.

In the flat plunge, which is used in shallow water, or where the depth is unknown, and which can be made only from a small height, the swimmer must fling himself forwards, in order to extend the line of the plunge as much as possible under the surface of the water; and, as soon as he touches it, he must keep his head up, his back hollow, and his hands stretched forward, flat and inclined upward.

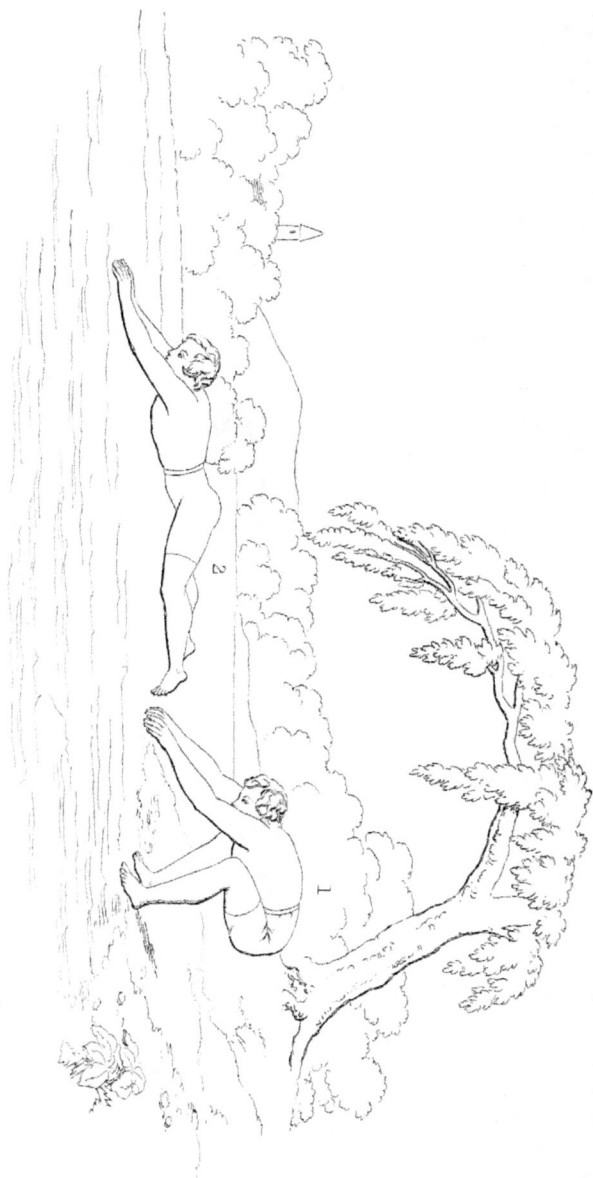

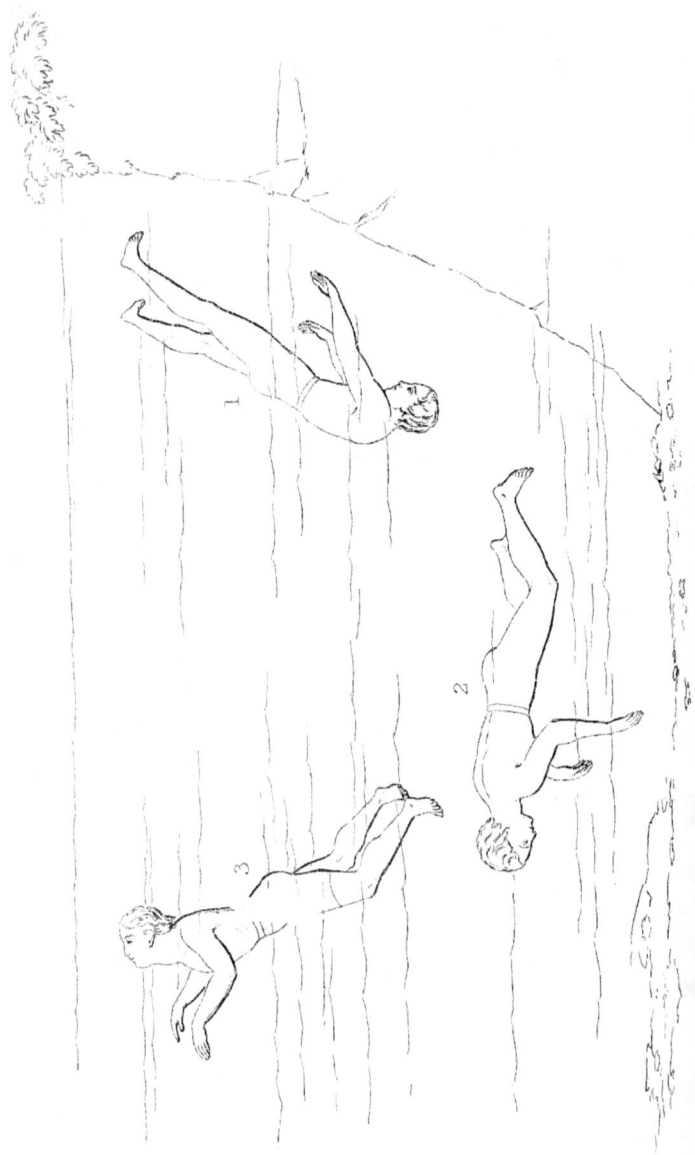

He will thus dart forwards a considerable way close under the surface, so that his head will reach it before the impulse ceases to operate. (Plate XXVI. fig. 2.)

DIVING.

The swimmer may prepare for diving by taking a slow and full inspiration, letting himself sink gently into the water, and expelling the breath by degrees, when the heart begins to beat strongly. In order to descend in diving, the head must be bent forward upon the breast; the back made round; and the legs thrown out with greater vigor than usual; but the arms and hands, instead of being struck forward as in swimming, must move rather backward, or come out lower, and pass more behind. (Plate XXVII. fig. 1.) The eyes should, meanwhile, be kept open, as, if the water be clear, it enables the driver to ascertain its depth, and see whatever lies at the bottom; and, when he has obtained a perpendicular position, he should extend his hands like feelers.

To move forward, the head must be raised, and the back straightened a little. Still, in swimming between top and bottom, the head must be kept a little downward, and the feet be thrown out a little higher than when swimming on the surface, (Plate XXVII. fig. 2;) and if the swimmer thinks that he approaches too near the surface, he must press the palms upwards. To ascend, the chin must be held up, the back made concave, the hands struck out high, and brought briskly down. (Plate XXVII. fig. 3.)

THRUSTING.

This is a transition from front swimming, in which the attitude and motions of the feet are still the same, but those of the hands very different. One arm, the right for

11*

instance, is lifted entirely out of the water, thrust forward
as much as possible, and, when at the utmost stretch, let
fall, with the hand hollowed, into the water, which it grasps
or pulls towards the swimmer in its return transversely towards the opposite arm-pit.　While the right arm is thus
stretched forth, the left, with the hand expanded, describes
a small circle to sustain the body, (Plate XXVIII. fig. 1;)
and, while the right arm pulls towards the swimmer, the
left, in a widely-described circle, is carried rapidly under
the breast, towards the hip.　(Plate XXVIII. fig. 2.)

When the left arm has completed these movements, it,
in its turn, is lifted from the water, stretched forward, and
pulled back,—the right arm describing first the smaller,
then the larger circle.　The feet make their movements
during the describing of the larger circle.　The thrust requires much practice; but, when well acquired, it not only
relieves the swimmer, but enables him to make great advance in the water, and is applicable to cases where rapidity
is required for a short distance.

SPRINGING.

Some swimmers, at every stroke, raise not only their neck
and shoulders, but breast and body, out of the water.　This,
when habitual, exhausts without any useful purpose.　As
an occasional effort, however, it may be useful in seizing
objects above; and it may then best be performed by the
swimmer drawing his feet as close as possible under his
body, stretching his hands forward, and, with both feet and
hands, striking the water strongly, so as to throw himself
out of it as high as the hips.

ONE-ARM SWIMMING.

Here the swimmer must be more erect than usual, hold

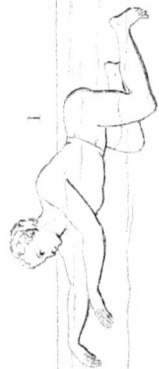

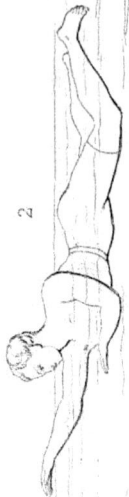

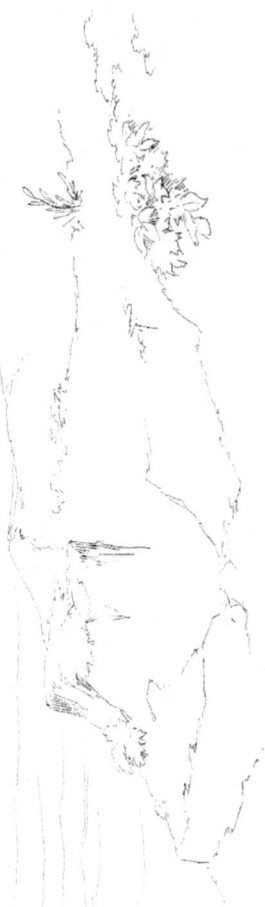

his head more backward, and use the legs and arm more quickly and powerfully. The arm, at its full extent, must be struck out rather across the body, and brought down before, and the breast kept inflated. This mode of swimming is best adapted for assisting persons who are drowning, and should be frequently practised—the learner carrying first under, then over the water, a weight of a few pounds.

In assisting drowning persons, however, great care should be taken to avoid being caught hold of by them. They should be approached from behind, and driven before, or drawn after the swimmer to the shore, by the intervention, if possible, of anything that may be at hand, and if nothing be at hand, by means of their hair; and they should, if possible, be got on their backs. Should they attempt to seize the swimmer, he must cast them loose immediately; and, if seized, drop them to the bottom, when they will endeavor to rise to the surface.

Two swimmers treading water may assist a drowning person by seizing him, one under each arm, and carrying him along with his head above water, and his body and limbs stretched out and motionless.

FEATS IN SWIMMING.

Men have been known to swim in their clothes a distance of 4000 feet.

Others have performed 2200 feet in twenty-nine minutes.

Some learn to dive and bring out of the water burdens as heavy as a man.

[This art, however, has made little if any progress from the earliest records that we possess of it. Leander's feat of passing from Abydos to Sestos, was the crack performance of antiquity; and it was the ultra achievement of

Lord Byron, probably one of the best swimmers of our day.—ED. Fifth Edition.]

ROWING.

RIVER ROWING,* WITH TWO SCULLS.

THE BOAT.

It may be laid down as a general rule, that, in calm weather, a light and sharp boat is preferable; and, in rough weather, a heavier and broader one. The learner, however, should not at first begin in too light a boat, nor should he practice in rough weather, until he gets acquainted with its management.

TO LEAVE THE LANDING-PLACE.

To leave the shore, the rower should, with the boat-hook, shove the boat off, head upon tide, or opposite to the current. To leave stairs, the rower must either shove the boat off with the boat-hook, or place the blade of the scull forward, and perform what the London watermen call belaying the boat's head out from the shore, accordingly as there is deep or shallow water.

This being done, the rower sits down to his sculls. These he puts in the rullocks, and turns the concave front, or filling of the scull, towards the stern of the boat.

THE SEAT.

The rower must sit a-midships on the thwart or seat of

* This should have the preference here, because the art is best learned on the smooth water, and in the lighter boats, of rivers.

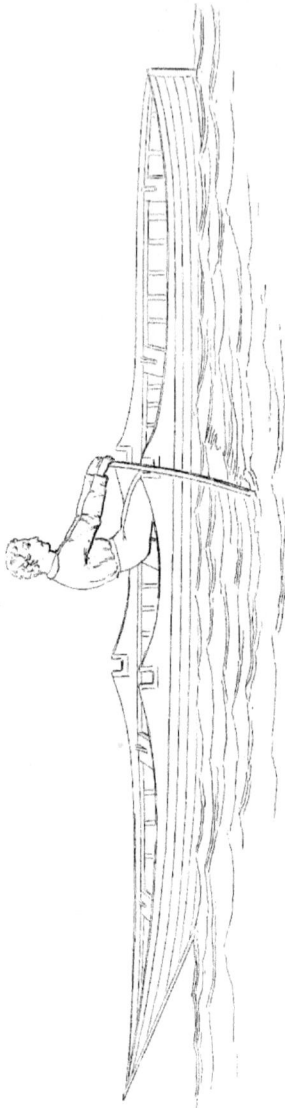

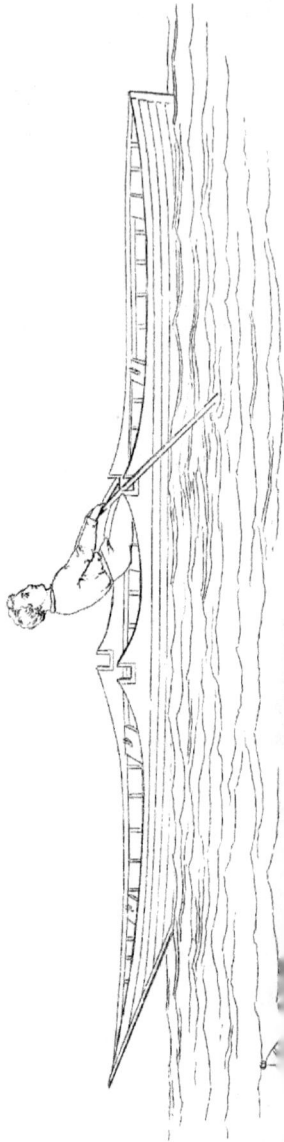

the boat, else she will heel to the side on which he is sitting, and much of his labor will be lost. He should sit with ease to himself, having his feet on the middle of the stretcher, and his legs not quite extended; but his knees, as he rows, should be brought down, and his legs stretched.

THE PULL.

The rower should make long strokes in a heavy boat, and shorter and quicker strokes in a light boat. At the beginning of the pull, he must, in general, bend his body till his head is over his knees, and extend his arms as far aft as convenient, that the blades of the sculls may be thrown correspondingly forward. (Plate XXIX. fig. 1.) With regard to the back in particular, some think that, if a short distance is to be rowed, it should be bent; and that if a long distance, it is less fatiguing to keep it straight. When the arms are extended as far aft, and the blades of the sculls as far forward as convenient—which must never be so far as to jam in the rullocks—(Plate XXIX. fig. 1.) the rower must dip the sculls into the water, and pull towards him, by at once bending the arms and the body.

When in the middle of the pull, if the sculls are not short enough, or even if the head and body are slightly turned, one of the hands will go higher than the other; and as the right is generally the stronger, it may go above, and the left below. It is often found difficult to keep one hand clear of the other in pulling a pair of sculls. This is so much the case, indeed, that the inexperienced frequently suffer more from the knocking and rubbing of the backs and sides of the hands against each other, than from the friction of the handles of the oars in the palms of the hands. This may be easily obviated by attending to the following advice :—

Having seated yourself in the centre of the thwart, with your feet close together against the centre of the stretcher, ship your sculls, but, before pulling a stroke, move your body three or four inches to the right hand, and still retain your feet in the centre : thus you will be sitting rather obliquely; this will throw your right shoulder more forward, and consequently the right hand ; and thus the hands will work perfectly clear of each other. This rule, however, must be modified by the circumstances of river-rowing.   A waterman writes us as follows :—As to carrying one hand above the other, my way is, that if, for instance, I go from Greenwich to Blackwall against tide, I keep down on the Greenwich side, in general look toward the shore, and having my face over the left shoulder, my right hand is then above.   If I go from Greenwich to London, my face is turned over the right shoulder, and the left hand is then uppermost."

(The usual position in the middle of the pull is shown in Plate XXIX. fig. 2.)

The end of the pull must not take place till the elbows have approached the tops of the hips, the hands are brought towards the chest, and the body is thrown well back. There would be a loss of power, however, if the hands were brought too near the chest; and the body should not be thrown further back than it may easily and quickly recover its first position for the next stroke.—(Plate XXX.)   As the water is being delivered from the sculls, the elbows sink, the wrists are bent up, and the backs of the hands are turned towards the fore-arms, in order to feather the sculls.—(Plate XXX. fig. 1.)

In the return of the sculls, the hands must remain turned up until the sculls are put into the water.—(Plate XXX. fig. 2.)   In the middle of the return, if the sculls are not short, or if the head and body be turned, one of the hands also goes higher than the other.

As to the degree of the immersion of the sculls.—In the middle of the pull, the blades must be covered by the water. The learner in general dips them very deep; but that ought to be avoided, especially in calm weather. In the whole of the return, the tips should, in calm weather, be two or three inches above the water; and, in rough weather, they should be higher, in order to clear it, as represented in the preceding plates. The head ought throughout to be very moveable—first to one side, then to the other, but generally turned towards the shore when against the tide. The same movements have only to be repeated, throughout the course.

THE TIDE OR CURRENT.

In river-rowing, when the tide or current is with the rower, a learner should in general take the middle of the stream. In rowing with the tide, however, watermen generally cut off the points, in order to keep a straight course. When the tide or current is against the rower, he should take the sides, preferring that side on which, owing to the course of the river, the current is least. As there is an eddy under the points, watermen generally, when rounding them, shoot the water to the next point, and so on.

TO TURN.

Back water with one scull, by putting the one on the side you wish to turn to into the water, with its concave front or filling towards you, and pushing against it; and at the same time pull strongly with the other scull, until the boat's head is turned round.

MEETING OR PASSING.

In meeting, the boat which comes with the tide must get out of the way. In this case, both boats, if close, lay the blades of their sculls flat on the water, lift them out of the rullocks, and let them drift alongside. Each replaces them when the other has passed. In passing a boat, the rower who passes must take the outside, unless there is ample room within, and must also keep clear of the other's sculls or oars. If one boat is crossing the water, and another coming with the tide, the one coming with tide must keep astern of the other, and have a good look-out ahead.

TO LAND.

Give the boat its proper direction, and keep its head inclining towards the tide, and its stern will turn up or down, as the tide runs; unship the sculls by the manœuvre directed above; but, instead of letting them drift alongside, lay them in the boat, the blades forward and the looms aft; seize the headfast; jump ashore; and take two half-hitches round the post or ring.

SEA-ROWING, OR ROWING IN A GALLEY ON THE RIVER.

In launching a boat from the sea-beach, when it is rough, and there is a heavy surf, the two bowmen must get into the boat with their oars run out; and the other rowers follow the boat quickly in her descent; but they should not jump in till she is quite afloat, lest their weight might fix her on the beach, and she might ship a sea.

It may happen that, immediately on the boat floating, a sea shall take the bow (before the rowers are sufficiently prepared with their oars to keep her head out), and place her broadside to the waves. In this situation, the boat is

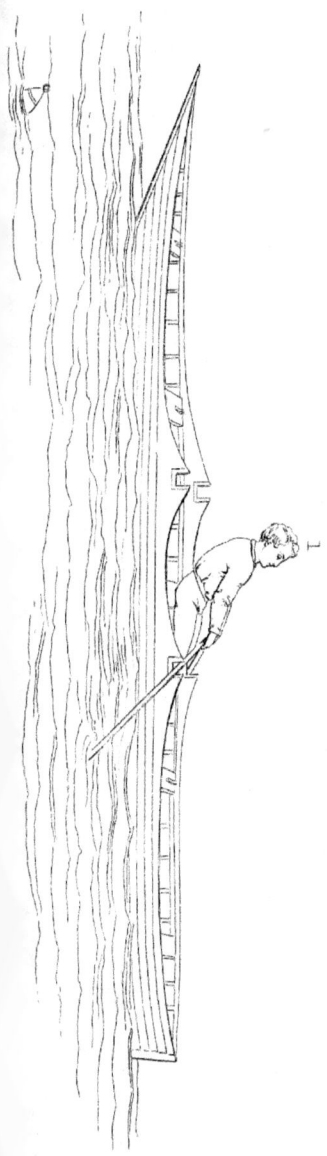

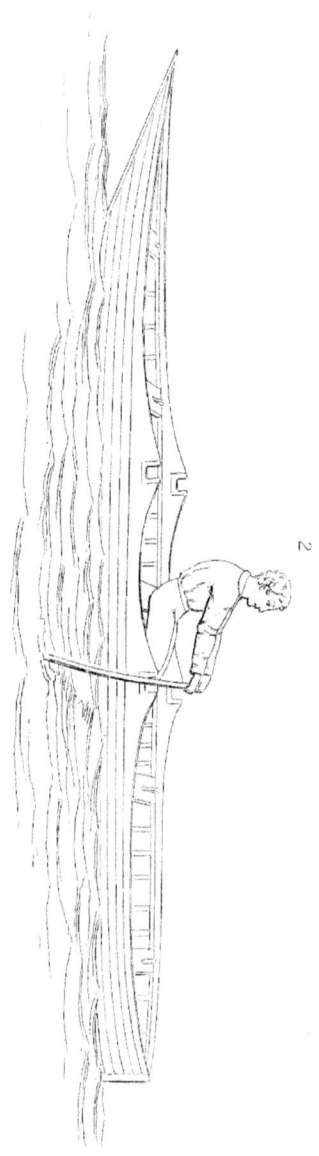

in danger of being swamped, and the lives of those on board are in peril. When thus situated, it is best for two of the rowers to go near the bow of the boat, and immediately force each his boat-hook or oar on the ground, on the shore side of the boat, as the most effectual, safe, and expeditious method of bringing her head again to the sea. Should there be more than a usual swell, both the rowers and the sitter, or steersman, cannot be too particular in keeping, throughout, the head of the boat to the swell, as lying broadside to a heavy sea is extremely dangerous.

In rowing, each man has in general a single oar, and sits on the opposite side of the galley from the rullock through which his oar passes. The oar must consequently cross the boat, and be held on its opposite side, so as to clear the back of the man before.

It should be neither held nor pulled obliquely to the side by twisting the body, as is practised by many, because the muscles in that case act disadvantageously, and are sooner fatigued. The stroke must be longer in sea than in river rowing. The oar must be thrown out with a heave, caused by the simultaneous extension of the body and the arms. It is still more essential to feather in sea than in river rowing.

The oar must be drawn back with great power, caused by the simultaneous contraction of the body and arms; time with the other rowers being accurately kept, and distinctly marked.

When the oars are delivered from the water, the time, until they go into it again, may be counted, one, two, three,—when they pass through the water. This time is kept by the strokesman, or sternmost man of the rowers.

In landing, the word is, "in bow," when the bowman or foremast man gets the boat-hook ready to clear away

12

for the shore, or the stairs. The next word is from the
coxwain, "rowed off all," or "well rowed;" when all the
oars are laid in, with the blades forward, and the boat is
made fast.

In landing on the sea beach, when there is a surf, the
rowers may watch for a smooth, and then give good way
ashore, when the bowman should instantly jump out with
the headfast or painter, and pull her up, to avoid shipping
a sea. The distances run in this way are very great. We
have known four men, in a short galley, row thirty miles
in four hours, namely, from Dover to eight miles below
Calais, or abreast of Gravelines, on the opposite coast. In
such a row, a London waterman would have no skin left
on his hands; and a member of the Funny Club would,
we suppose, have no hands left on his arms!

SAILING.

BOATS, ETC.

Cutters, owing to their excellent sailing qualities, are
much employed as packets,* revenue cruisers, smugglers,
privateers, and in all cases requiring despatch. The boats
commonly employed in parties of pleasure, &c., are also
cutters.

On the size of these vessels, however, it is necessary to
remark, that a cutter under one hundred tons is sufficiently
handy; but, when the size is equal to that of the larger
yachts, a strong crew is necessary, as the spars are very
heavy, and a number of men requisite to set or shorten
sail. As a single-masted vessel, in the event of springing
a spar, becomes helpless, even large cutters are used only

* In the packet line, since the general adoption of steam, cutters are
seldom if ever met with.—ED. Fifth Edition.

in short voyages, or on the coast; for, in case of accident, they can always manage to reach some harbor or anchorage to repair any damage they may sustain. The peculiar qualities of beating well to windward, and working on short tacks, adapt cutters peculiarly for channel cruising.

Although, some years back, large cutters were confined principally to the navy and revenue, the Royal Yacht Squadron, in theirs, have exceeded these not only in size, but in beauty and sailing qualities. Some of the finest and fastest cutters in the world are the property of this national club; and two of them, the Alarm (Mr. Weld's), and the Arundel* (the Duke of Norfolk's), measure 193 and 188 tons. The inconvenient size, however, of a cutter's boom and mainsail has caused the very general introduction of a ketch rig, which, by the addition of a mizen, permits the boom to be dispensed with, and reduces the mainsail considerably. This rig, indeed, when the mizen stands well, is elegant; and, if a vessel is short-handed, it is very handy. As cutter-rigged vessels, instead of a regular mainsail, with its boom and gaff, have sometimes a mere spritsail, it is necessary we should observe, that the inferior convenience and safety of these preclude our noticing them here. It is also necessary that we should explain why, in the sequel, we do not even refer to lugger-rigged vessels.

Luggers are more difficult to work or manœuvre; they require a greater number of men; their spars are so heavy that they require all hands to move them; their decks are inevitably lumbered with spars, &c.; their canvass gets rotted from exposure; and their expense is much greater

---

* The tonnage of the Arundel is not given here according to the Royal Yacht Squadron list: there it is stated to be 210 tons.—ED. Fifth Edition.

than that of cutters. They generally have two sets of lugs —large ones, which require dipping every time they tack, and small working lugs, which do not require dipping, the tack coming to the foot of the mast. The latter are generally used, except in making long reaches across the channel, &c. A lugger, moreover, is seldom fit to be altered to anything but a schooner, not having breadth enough for one mast, which, after all, is the best for beauty and speed.

Sailing men, indeed, are now so perfectly aware of the inferior speed of luggers, that we never see a lugger or schooner enter against a cutter at all near its tonnage. At sea, luggers would have a better chance; though even there many would prefer cutters, except in foul weather and a long reach. In short, these vessels suit only a few noblemen and gentlemen who have enough of patriotic ambition to desire to look like smugglers, enough of delicacy to disregard the being thought dirty lubbers by their own men—some of whom are not dirty from mere taste or choice, and enough of penetration not to discover, that on their landing with filthy clothes and tarry hands, every old sailor grins or laughs at their imagining, that it was they, and not the man at the helm, who had kept the canvass from cracking, or the sticks from going over the side. Our descriptions apply, therefore, to cutters alone; and the plates at the end of this article illustrate the various parts therein referred to.

Upon the Thames, the sailing clubs comprise the Royal Sailing Society, the Royal Thames Yacht Club, the Loyal Victoria Yacht Club, the Clarence, British, Royal Yacht, and several minor associations. Several cups and prizes are annually given during the season; and the spirited contests between the beautiful small craft which form these fancy fleets, are highly interesting. The sailing matches on the river are of two sorts—one above, and the other below the bridges. The smaller yachts, of from six to twenty-six tons, are commonly entered for the former, and a larger class for the latter, which take place between Greenwich and Gravesend. These national amusements appear to be rapidly gaining the first place among fashionable recreations, and now occupy the season, from the period when hunting ends, till shooting begins.

The Royal Yacht Squadron has nearly six hundred persons on its lists, of which above one hundred are members, and about four hundred and fifty honorary members. The number of yachts is one hundred and nine;* of which eighty-seven are cutters, ten schooners, three brigs, four yawls, two ships, two ketches, and one lugger. The greater part of these vessels hail from Cowes or Southampton. The shipping belonging to the club amounts to 7250 tons. Now, a vessel of one hundred tons seldom perhaps stands the owner in less than from five to six thousand pounds, varying from that to ten, according to the profusion of ornamental parts, the internal fittings, and other contingencies. At this rate, the shipping of the club would have cost more than three millions and a half of money: but it is impossible to speak decisively on this point, as the first cost of the yachts varies much, and the numerous styles of rig are attended with expenses so widely different. At a moderate computation, each vessel belonging to the club carries ten men on an average : this gives the total number employed 1090. During the summer months, then, while regattas are celebrated, it may be said that the Royal Yacht Squadron alone employs more than 1100 men. These,

* As the number is constantly fluctuating, we had better take the average at a hundred, which will be found quite as high a one as we should be justified in suggesting.

with some few exceptions, are discharged on the approach of winter, and the yachts are laid up for the season, retaining the master and one man in pay. The crews thus discharged obtain employment in merchant vessels, or otherwise, during the winter; and in the middle of spring are generally re-shipped in the yachts in which they have previously served. On these conditions, active and industrious men of good character are generally sure of employment in the club; and many members justly pride themselves on the high discipline, manly bearing, and crack appearance of their crews. The situation of master, in particular, is one of much responsibility, and is on all accounts respectably filled. In some of the largest craft, junior officers of the navy are found to accept this office. The sailing regulations of the Royal Yacht Squadron are as follows;

First—Members entering their yachts must send the names of them to the secretary, one week previous to the day of sailing, and pay two guineas entrance at the same time.

Second—All vessels starting or entering must be the *bonâ fide* property of members, as well as their spars, sails, boats, &c.

Third—Each member is allowed to enter one vessel only for all prizes given by the club.

Fourth—Cutters may carry four sails only, viz., mainsail, foresail, jib, and gaff top-sail; yawls, luggers, schooners, and all other vessels, in like proportion. No booming out allowed.

Fifth—No trimming with ballast, or shifting of ballast allowed; and all vessels to keep their platforms down, and bulkheads standing.

Sixth—Vessels on the larboard tack must invariably

give way to those on the starboard tack; and in all cases where a doubt of the possibility of the vessel on the larboard tack weathering the one on the starboard tack shall exist, the vessel on the larboard tack shall give way; or, if the other vessel keep her course, and run into her, the owner of the vessel on the larboard tack shall be compelled to pay all damages, and forfeit his claim to the prize.

Seventh—Vessels running on shore shall be allowed to use their own anchors and boats actually on board, to get them off, afterwards weighing anchor and hoisting the boat in; but, upon receiving assistance from any other vessel or vessels, boats, or anchors, shall forfeit all claim to the prize.

Eighth—That nothing but the hand-line be used for sounding.

Ninth—Any deviation from these rules shall subject the aggressor to forfeit all claim to the prize.

Tenth—If any objection be made with regard to the sailing of any other vessel in the race, such objection must be made to the stewards, within one hour after the vessel making the objection arrive at the starting-post.

Eleventh—No vessel shall be allowed to take in ballast, or take out, for twenty-four hours previous to starting; and no ballast shall be thrown overboard.

Twelfth—Vessels shall start from moorings laid down at a cable-length distance, with their sails set; and every vessel not exceeding one hundred tons shall carry a boat not less than ten feet long; and vessels exceeding one hundred tons, a boat not less than fourteen feet long.

Thirteenth—There shall be a member, or honorary member, on board each vessel.

Fourteenth—The time of starting may be altered by the stewards; and all disputes that may arise are to be decided by them, or such persons as they shall appoint.

The Northern Yatch Club is a highly interesting society, although its plan is not so extensive as that of the Royal Club. It contains about three hundred and fifty members. The documents for 1830 comprise ninety-two in the Scottish, and ninety in the Irish division, with fifty-two honorary members, in addition to ninety-three members of the Cork Yacht Club, who are also entered on the honorary lists. It had, in 1830, sixty yachts, not equal in proportion to the tonnage of the Cowes Club, as smaller vessels are admitted. Many R. Y. S. men are found in the Northern Club. There are many fine vessels in this Club. Cutters, as usual, excel in number.

At the lowest computation, the number of vessels at present employed for pleasure in this country cannot be less than from three to four hundred, ranging in bulk from ten to three hundred and fifty tons. These are variously distributed along our shores, carrying their opulence into every port and harbor. But there is another advantage arising from the yacht clubs—namely, that national spirit, which, to a maritime people, is above all in worth. The yacht clubs keep alive this feeling in an eminent degree.

COURSES, ETC.

Even in describing the elementary nautical operations which such boats require, it is necessary to lay down a position for the HARBOR, direction for the WIND, and trip for the VESSEL.

Let us suppose, then, that the mouth of the harbor lies toward the south ; that the wind blows from the north, with a little inclination to east, and that we wish first to sail due south to get out of the harbor, next direct our course eastward, then return westward till we get abreast the mouth of the harbor, and lastly, northward, to enter the harbor and come to our moorings.

These courses will, with variations in the force of the wind, illustrate every common and useful manœuvre.

GETTING UNDER WAY.

Ship* the tiller.†

Set the mainsail;‡ hoist the throat§ nearly close up; and half hoist the peak.||

Bend¶ and haul the jib out to the bowsprit end.

Bowse the bobstay** and bowsprit shrouds†† well taut.

Hoist the jib, and bowse it well up.

Get the topmast stay,‡‡ backstays,§§ and rigging|||| well taut.

* Fix in its proper place.

† The piece of wood or beam put into the head of the rudder to move it.

‡ Unfurl it by casting the stops or gaskets off.

§ The foremost end of the gaff, or that end next the mast.

|| The outermost end of the gaff, or that farthest from the mast.

¶ Hook it to the traveller, or ring on the bowsprit.

**A rope or chain from the end of the bowsprit to half-way down the stem.

†† Ropes from the bowsprit end on each side to the bows.

‡‡ A rope from the topmast head to the outer end of the bowsprit, where it passes through a sheave or small block, comes in by the stem head, and is belayed or made fast (done generally by winding several times backwards and forwards in the manner of a figure 8,) to its cleat or pin.

§§ Ropes from the after-part of the head of the topmast to the after-part of the channels on each side.

|||| Or shrouds—ropes from each side of the topmast head, through the cross-tree arms, to the fore part of the channels, between the first and second lower shroud. They are set up or hauled taut, as are the backstays, by means of a small tackle, one block of which is hooked to the thimble spliced into the lower end of the shroud or backstay, and the other to an eye-bolt in the channels.

Hoist the foresail ready to cast* her when the moorings are let go.

Send a hand to the helm.†

Overhaul the main-sheet,‡ and the lee§ runner and tackle;‖ lower the throat, and hoist the peak of the mainsail taut¶ up.

Hoist the gaff topsail,** keeping the tack†† to windward‡‡ of the peak halyards,§§ and hauling the slack of the sheet out before you hoist the sail taut up.

Set the tack, and heave the sheet well taut.

BEFORE THE WIND.‖‖

With the Main Boom over to Starboard.¶¶

In managing the helm, be careful not to jibe the main-sail.

* To turn her head in the most advantageous direction.

† This term includes both the tiller and the wheel; but, as the yawing motion of a small light vessel is correspondingly light and feeble, though much quicker than that of a large vessel, she is best without a wheel, which is meant to gain power at the expense of time.

‡ A rope or tackle for regulating the horizontal position of the main boom.

§ The leeward or lee-side is the opposite to windward.

‖ A compound tackle, used in cutter-rigged vessels, instead of a backstay to the lower mast, on account of its easy removal allowing the main boom to go forward, in going large.

¶ The nautical way of pronouncing and writing *tight*.

** The sail above the mainsail. The sheet hauls out to a small block on the outer end of the gaff.

†† Tack is the lowermost corner opposite to the sheet, in all fore-and-aft sails and studding sails.

‡‡ The windward or weather side, is that side on which the wind blows.

§§ The rope by which the peak of the gaff or boom, to which the head of the mainsail is fastened, is hoisted. Halyards always signifies a rope by which a sail is hoisted.

‖‖ That is, going the same way the wind blows. Her course is then sixteen points from the wind. (See Compass.)

¶¶ Starboard is the right, and larboard the left-hand side, when looking toward the head of the vessel.

When a vessel is going large,* the helmsman should always place himself on the weather side of the tiller, or the side opposite to that which the main boom is over, as his view of the vessel's head will then be unobstructed by the sails. The boat now running before the wind, haul the tack of mainsail up. If the wind come dead aft, you may flatten aft the jib and foresail sheets,† or haul the foresail down to prevent chafing. If the wind come at all round on the starboard quarter,‡ slack off the boom guy;§ haul in the main-sheet till you get the boom a-midships,|| or nearly so; port¶ the helm, and jibe the mainsail; slack off the main-sheet again, and hook the guy on the larboard side; haul taut the starboard runner and tackle, and overhaul the larboard one; the same with the topping-lift;** hoist the head sails,†† and shift the sheets over.

---

* Or free, not close-hauled. Generally understood as having the wind abaft the beam, or that her course is then eight points from the wind.

† Ropes fast to the aftermost lower corner of the jib and foresail, to hold them down. The jib has two ropes or sheets fast to its corner, one of which comes on each side the forestay, for the convenience of tacking, &c. The foresail has only one sheet, which is fast to the traveller, or ring on the horse or bar of iron, which crosses from one gunwale to the other, just before the mast.

‡ The point on either side where the side and stern meet.

§ A small tackle, one end of which is hooked to the main boom, and the other forward, to keep the boom from swinging.

|| Midway between the sides of the vessel.

¶ Instead of larboard, when speaking of the helm, port is the proper term, in contrariety to starboard, used for the sake of distinctness in directing the helmsman.

** Stout ropes which lead, one from each side the main boom near its outer end, through a block on its respective side the mast, just under the cross-trees, whence it descends about half-way, and is connected to the deck or gunwale by a tackle.

†† Jib and foresail.

N. B. If you are obliged to jibe as above, you must, in the following directions for bringing the wind on your beam, read larboard for starboard, and *vice versâ*.

BRINGING THE VESSEL WITH THE WIND ON THE LARBOARD BEAM.*

Supposing that you have not jibed, starboard the helm a little, and let the vessel spring her luff† with her head to the northward. Slack the boom guy, and haul in the main-sheet. Haul aft‡ the jib-sheet, and bowline§ the foresail.

If she come up fast, port the helm‖ a little, and meet her; then right¶ it when she lays her proper course.

Hook and haul taut the lee runner and tackle. You will now find it necessary to carry the helm a little a-port or a-weather.

––––––

If, instead of directing our course eastward, we had preferred doing so westward, we must have jibed previous to bringing the wind on the beam, and then the preceding operations would necessarily have been, to a corresponding extent, reversed.

* That is, athwart or across the waist of the vessel, called a-beam, because it is in the same direction that her beams lay, or at right angles with her keel. Her head is then eight points from the wind.— The wind is said to be abaft the beam, or before the beam, according as the vessel's head is more or less than eight points from the wind.

† Sail nearer to the wind.

‡ That is, toward the hinder part or stern.

§ A rope made fast to the foremost shroud, and passed through a thimble in the after-leach of the foresail, then round the shroud again, and round the sheet.

‖ Always put the helm the contrary way to that which you want the vessel's head to turn.

¶ That is, bring it amidships; the same with *steady*.

CLOSE-HAULING THE VESSEL.*

To haul the vessel to the wind, ease the helm down† a little. Haul in the main-sheet upon the proper mark. Bowse the fore-sheet, and haul the jib-sheet well aft. Bowse the runner and tackle well taut.

The vessel is now on the wind, plies to windward, or is close-hauled.‡

Being now apt to gripe, or come up into the wind with a sudden jerk, now and again, she will carry her helm more or less a-weather. The helmsman must watch the weather-leach of the mainsail, to prevent the vessel getting her head in the wind.

TACKING.§

Having got abreast or opposite the mouth of the harbor, haul the fore bowline. "Ready about."‖ Put your helm up, or to windward a little, and let the vessel go rather off the wind, to get good way on her, then gently down or to

---

* To haul the sheets aboard, or more amidships, by which means the vessel's head will come closer to the point the wind blows from.

† To leeward.

‡ These terms all imply one thing, viz., that the vessel is sailing as near as possible to the point whence the wind blows. No square-rigged vessel will sail within less than six, and no fore-and-aft rigged vessel within less than five, points of the wind, to have any headway.

§ To turn a vessel from one side to the other with her head toward the wind. When a vessel is obliged to tack several times successively to get to windward, she is said to be beating to windward; when to get up or down a harbor, channel, &c., beating up or down, &c.; when trying to get off a lee shore, clawing off.

A vessel's tacks are always to windward and forward; and her sheets to leeward and aft; whence the terms larboard or starboard tack, meaning that she has her tacks aboard on the larboard or starboard side.

‖ A command that all hands are to be attentive, and at their stations for tacking.

leeward with it, which is announced by the helmsman calling "Helm's a-lee." Let fly the jib-sheet: this takes off the balance of wind from her head, and acts in concert with the helm in sweeping her stern to leeward, or rather in allowing her head to come quicker up into the wind.

The man who attends the jib-sheet must carefully gather in the slack* of the one opposite to that which he let go. When the jib comes over the larboard side of the stay,† haul the larboard jib-sheet well aft. When the mainsail is filled, let draw the foresail.‡ Right the helm, and shift over the tack of the mainsail.

One hand should attend the main sheet, to gather in the slack till the boom is amidships, and then ease it off as the sail fills, and the vessel lays over to port. When the vessel is in stays, and it is doubtful whether she will come round, or, in order to make her come round when she gathers stern-way, shift the helm to the opposite side. She is now about upon the starboard tack.

REEFING, TAKING IN SAIL, ETC.

Haul the fore-sheet up to windward; bowline it there, and heave her to. Keep the tiller shipped, and lash it a-lee. In gaff topsail; lower the halyards; and haul down. Send a hand aloft to unbend the sheet from the sail, and

* Or loose rope.

† The forestay, or large rope from the lower mast head to the stem head, to prevent the mast from springing when the vessel is sending deep, or fallen into the hollow between two waves, after pitching.

‡ That is, let go the bowline which holds the sail to this, now weather shroud. It was held there till now, that the wind might act upon it with greater power to turn the vessel, from the time her head was about half way round. The expression is derived from its being necessary, in larger vessels of a similar rig, to ease the rope gradually as the sail draws it. From the time the jib-sheet is let fly, till the foresail is let draw, the vessel is said to be *in stays*.

make it fast to the main halyard bolt; and unlash the gaff topsail, and send it down. Lower the main halyards and peak to the second reef cringle, and reef the mainsail.

Hook the reef tackle* to the first earing;† haul upon it till the cringle‡ is close down upon the boom; and belay the tackle. Pass a small gasket§ through the tack and the first reef cringle, and lash the two firmly together, taking care to gather in snug the luff of the sail, so that the leach rope belonging to it forms a sort of snake near the mast. Haul up the tack, and bowse upon the weather peak line, keeping the other part fast amidships of the boom. This will hold the belly of the sail partly to windward, and make it easier to tie the reef-points. Observe to keep the foot-rope outside and under the sail.

Let one man jump upon the boom to tie the outer points so far that the rest can be tied on board. Let go the tack and peak line, always keeping the ends of this fast under the boom. Hoist the sail taut up; and set taut the tack tackle. Shift the jib to No. 2. Overhaul the jib purchase; let go the outhaul; haul the jib down; unhook the tack; unbend the sheets: and send the sail down below.

* A small tackle formed of two hook blocks, one of which is hooked to the under part of the boom, about one-third from the mast, and the other farther aft. The fall is belayed to a cleat under the boom.

† A stout rope, one end of which is made fast to the boom at the same distance from the mast as the reef cringle to which it belongs. It ascends, passes through the cringle, descends and passes through a sheave on the side of the boom, then in board, and is stopped to the boom by means of its lanyard, or small line spliced into its end for the purpose. This lanyard is also to make it fast when the sail is reefed, and you wish to remove the tackle.

‡ A short loop of rope with a thimble or small ring of iron inside it, spliced to the leach of the sail.

§ A rope made by plaiting rope-yarns.

You have now got one reef in the mainsail. If it come on to blow harder, and you want a second reef, lower the sail, and haul on the peak line as before; nipper the first reef-earing so as to hold it a short time; let go the reef tackle, and unhook it from the earing, which make fast with its lanyard round the boom.

You have now got the tackle to use for the second reef. Proceed as for the first reef. Shift the jib to No. 3, and proceed as before. If third, the same, after rigging the bowsprit. Take the fid* or bolt out of the heel of the bowsprit, and rig the bowsprit in about one fid hole. Haul taut the topmast stay and bowsprit rigging. Bend and set the small jib in the same way as any other.

You may want to stow the mainsail, set the trysail, and make her otherwise snug in proportion. Sway away upon the top rope; lift the mast a little to let the man unfid it; and lower topmast down in the slings. Lower the fore halyards, and reef the foresail. Gather the luff of the sail up; make the foremost reef-earing cringle fast to the tack; shift the sheet from the clue of the sail to the after reef cringle; and tie the points. If the weather is very heavy, haul down the stay-sail, and tend the vessel with a tackle upon the weather jib-sheet.

When it comes fine weather again, make sail in precisely the reverse order to that in which you shorten it. Continue to tack in the wind's eye till you are to windward of the harbor.

* A bar of wood or iron, which passes horizontally through a hole in each bitt and the heel of the bowsprit, to secure it in its place, much in the same way that a carriage pole is secured.

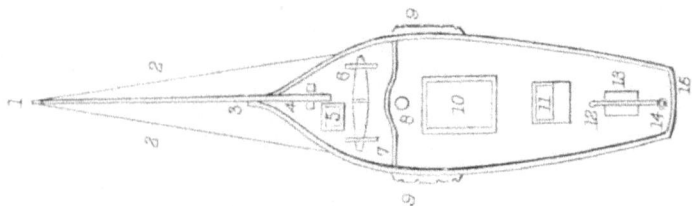

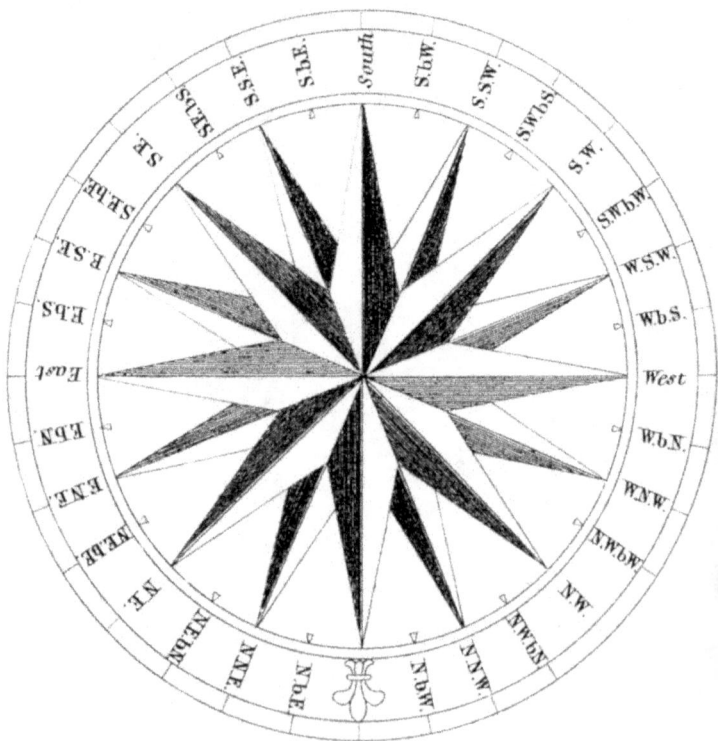

PASSING OTHER VESSELS.

All vessels sailing before the wind keep out of the way of those upon the wind. In the river Thames, vessels which sail with the larboard tack aboard, keep away for those with the starboard tack aboard.

BRINGING THE VESSEL INTO HARBOR.

Lower and haul down the gaff topsail. Let go the jib tack or outhaul;* lower the jib; and pull on the downhauler, to bring the traveller in. Haul the tack of the mainsail up; and lower the peak. Down foresail.

Let a small boat run away the wrap to the quay. Lower, and stow the mainsail. Unbend the jib, and stow it below if dry and not immediately wanted, and hook the halyards to the traveller, close in by the stem. If otherwise, hoist upon the halyards, and let it hang to dry if it require it, or stop it up and down the foremost shroud. Haul the vessel to the moorings, and moor properly, putting fenders over to keep her from the quay.

DESCRIPTION OF PLATE XXXI.

Fig. 1.

The mariner's compass.

Fig. 2.

Plan of the deck, with the bowsprit rigged out, &c.

1. Bowsprit.
2. 2. Bowsprit shrouds.
3. Stem head.
4. Bowsprit bitts.
5. Fore hatchway.
6. Windlass and bitts.

* A rope made fast to the traveller, to haul it out to the bowsprit end.

13*

7. Fore-sheet horse.
8. Place of the mast.
9. 9. Channels.
10. Main hatchway.
11. Companion and binnacle.

12 Tiller.
13. Cabin skylight.
14. Rudder-head and case.
15. Taffrail.

PLATE XXXII. fig. 1.

Pleasure boat, cutter-rigged, lying at anchor; foresail and mainsail bent and stowed.

1. Vane and spindle.
2. Truck.
3. Topmast.
4. Cap.
5. Trussel trees.
6. Lower mast.
7. 7. Cross trees.
8. Bowsprit.
9. Gaff, with mainsail furled.
10. Main boom.
11. Tiller.
12. Rudder.
13. Stem.
14. 14. Topmost shrouds.
15. Topmost backstay.

16. Topmost stay.
17. Runner and tackle.
18. Traveller.
19. Channel.
20. Forestay with the foresail furled to it.
21. Bobstay.
22. Topping-lifts.
23. Topping-lift blocks.
24. Main-sheet.
25. 25. Peak halyards.
26. Jib halyards.
27. Cable.
28. Fore-sheet.

PLATE XXXII. fig. 2.

The vessel going down the harbor with all sails set, steering south, before a light breeze.

1. Gaff topsail.
2. Foresail.
3. Mainsail.
4. Tack tricing line.
5. Peak line, or signal halyards.
6. 7. 8. The 1st, 2d, and 3d reefs.
9. 9. 9. Reef-earings.

10. 10. 10. Cringles.
11. Balance reef.
12. Anchor stock.
13. Windlass.
14. Foresheet horse.
15. Main hatch.
16. Companion and binnacle.

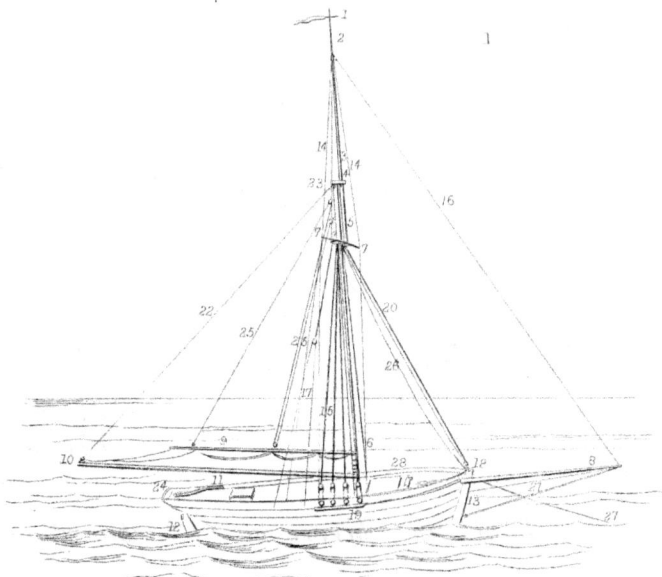

Parts in Pleasure Boat at Anchor

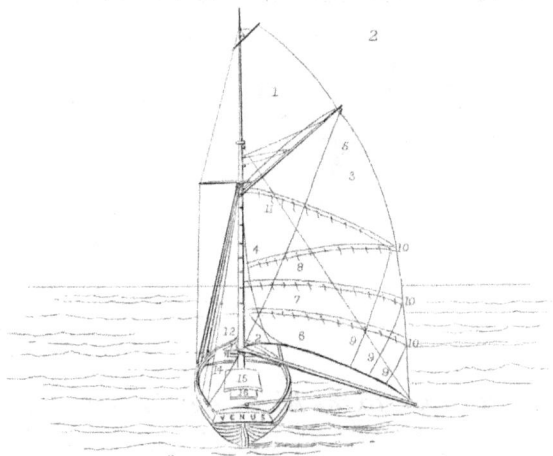

Boat before a light Breeze

Plate XXXIII

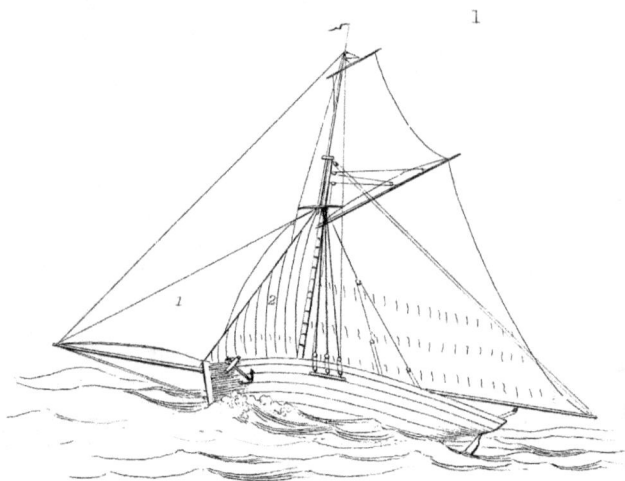

Boat with a breeze on the larboard beam

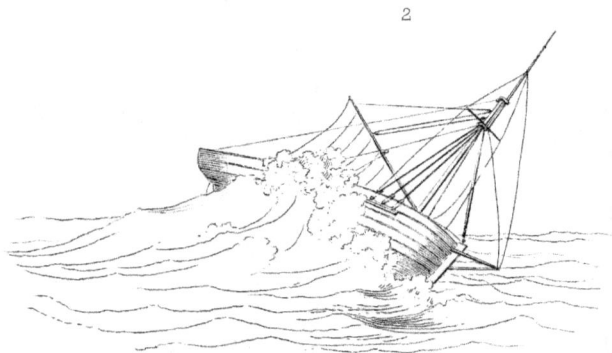

Boat close to the Wind on the Starboard tack

PLATE XXXIII. fig. 1.

The vessel outside the harbor, stearing east, with a smart breeze on the larboard beam.

1. Jib.	3. Anchor.
2. Foresail.	4. Eyebolt of the bowsprit shrouds.

PLATE XXXIII. fig. 2.

The vessel trying for the harbor in a heavy gale, close to the wind as she can lay, on the starboard tack, under a reefed mainsail and foresail, bowsprit reefed, and topmast lowered.

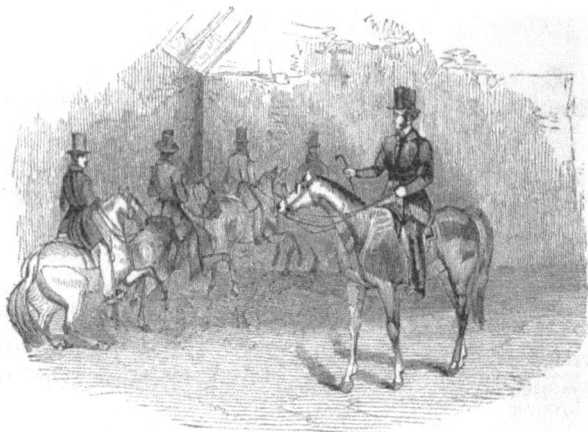

RIDING.

THE general art of riding, sometimes called manège riding, to distinguish it from its modifications in road-riding, hunting, racing, &c., teaches us to place every part of the body so that it can act upon the horse in every emergency, shows the effect of all the aids or modes of guiding him, and enables us to render him obedient to the slightest touch. By never suffering the ascendency to be transferred to the horse, by in general preventing him from making all his speed, and by exhausting him the sooner the more he exerts himself without permission, it bestows upon the rider perfect security.

An intimate knowledge of this method is necessary even to our abandoning it when convenient, to our adopting the styles, afterwards to be described, for more extended and rapid paces, or for long continued riding, to our suffering the horse to take more or less of ascendency, and to our, when necessary, easily recovering that superiority of the

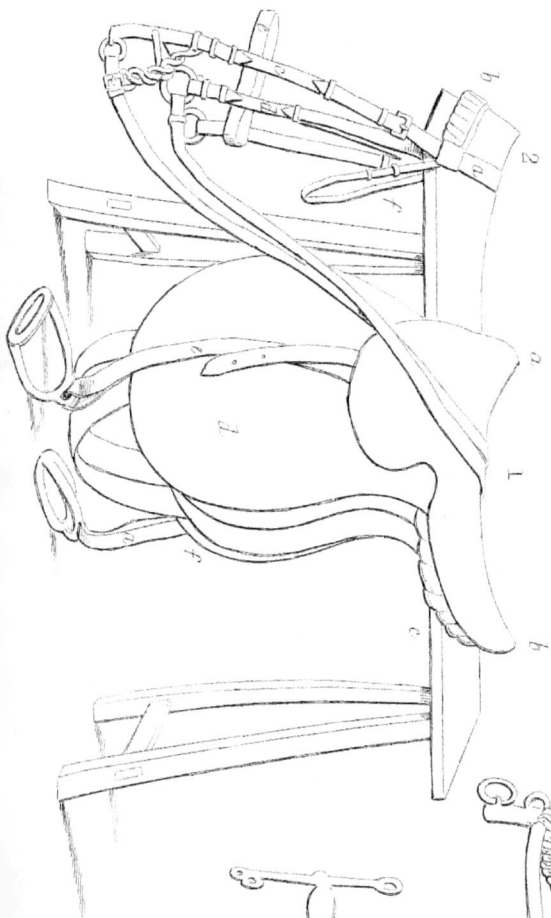

Plate XXXV

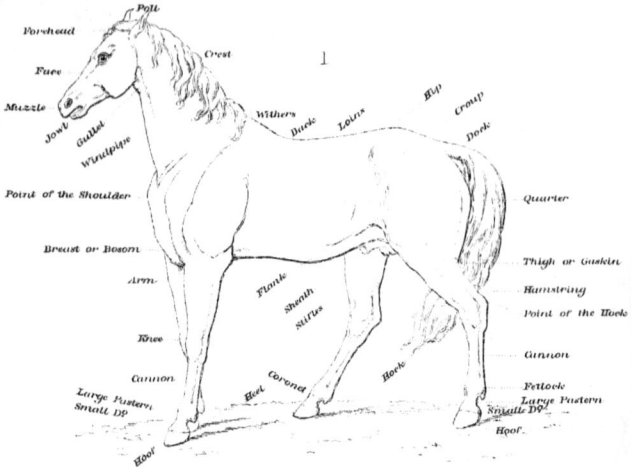

Poll
Forehead
Face
Crest
Muzzle
Jowl
Gullet
Windpipe
Withers
Back
Loins
Hip
Croup
Dock
Point of the Shoulder
Quarter
Breast or Bosom
Thigh or Gaskin
Arm
Flank
Hamstring
Sheath
Stifle
Point of the Hock
Knee
Gammon
Cannon
Coronet
Fetlock
Large Pastern,
Heel
Hock
Large Pastern
Small D?
Small D?
Hoof
Hoof

The Parts of the Horse

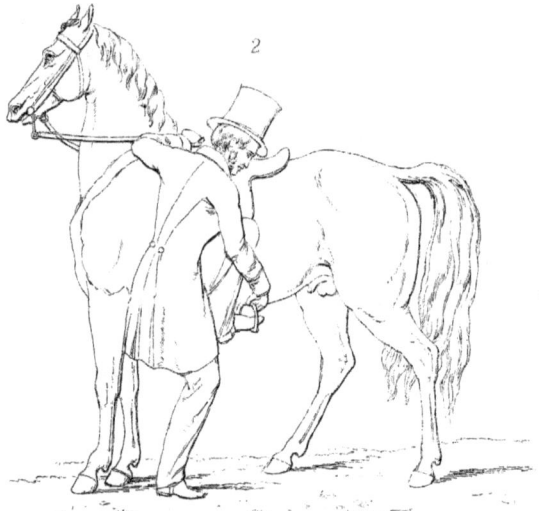

First View of Mounting

hand, of which those who are ignorant of this fundamental method are less capable.

The recent practice has been to carry the foot rather more forward than is represented in our Plates, approaching in this respect, to the ancient position, as seen in the Elgin marbles, &c.

A Parisian bit, which is attached to the mouth of the horse, without a headstall, has been lately used. It is, however, applicable only to *horses*, on account of its being retained in the mouth by means of the side tusks, which *mares* do not possess. It is composed of a semicircular bar of iron, which goes under the chin, to which its concavity applies; while a short bar, firmly attached to one of its ends, passes nearly half-way through the mouth. Through the other end of the semicircle is a hole, into which, when the bit is on, must be screwed a bolt, similar to the one just described. These two bolts, it is easily understood, pass behind the tusks, and nearly meet in the centre of the mouth.*

THE HORSE AND EQUIPMENTS.

Plates XXXIV. XXXV. fig. 1, give better ideas of the horse and his equipments than the longest and most detailed description. The reader will therefore examine them in succession. We have here only to add those cir-

---

* THE SADDLE (*Fig.* 1.)—*a*, pommel; *b*, cantle; *c*, pannel; *d*, flaps; *e*, stirrup leather; *f*, girths.

BRIDLES (*Fig.* 2.)—*a, b*, headstall with the chéek-straps; *c*, do. of the curb; *d*, do. of the bridoon or snaffle passing through it over the poll; *e*, nosetrap (seldom found in any but military bridles,) *f*, throatlash. *Fig.* 3. A twisted snaffle-bit. *Fig.* 4. A plain snaffle-bit. *Fig.* 5. A Weymouth curb, with chain and chain-strap (*a*) attached. *Fig.* 6. A common curb-bit, with the upset in the mouth-piece.

cumstances as to the equipment of the horse, which could not be communicated by that otherwise briefer and more impressive method.

The shoes of a horse have much to do with this, and consequently with his rider's comfort. It is therefore important to know that he is properly shod. To effect this, the shoe should be fitted to the foot, and not the foot to the shoe.

Neither heel nor frog should be pared more than merely to take off what is ragged; for no reproduction takes place here, as in the case of the hoof. Farriers ruin nearly all horses by doing otherwise. Indeed, they are not to be trusted with this operation, which, after shoeing, any gentleman may perform with his pocket-knife. The sole of the foot must not be hollowed out, but only the outer wall pared flat or even with the sole, and most at the toe. Nor, above all things, ought the farrier's finishing rasp all round the edge of the horn immediately above the shoe to be permitted. Neither ought nails to be driven far backward towards the heel, where the horn is softer and more sensible, especially of the inner quarter. When a horse has a high heel, the foot, except the frog, may be pared flat, but not hollowed out or opened. When a horse has a low heel, the foot should be pared only at the toes.

It is common to allow the fore part or toe of the hoof to grow long, thereby throwing the horse much on his heels. This position is unnatural, because, were the horse in a state of nature, without shoes, the toe, from constant contact with the ground, would be worn down to its proper level with the heel. This growth, then, of the fore part of the hoof, by throwing him on his heels, renders them tender, and causes lameness: while the foot, not being flat on the ground, also strains the ligaments of the fetlock joint. These evils may be obviated by doing as nature directs—by cutting away the toe to the proper level with the heel, so as to allow the foot to bear flat upon the ground. When a horse has a short pastern, he should have a short shoe, because a long one would compel him to bring his heel more backward than the unpliableness of his pastern would easily admit.

The saddle should be proportioned to the size of the horse. Before, the bearings should be clear of the plate bone; behind, they should not extend further than within four inches of the hips; and their pressure should be equal on every part intended to be touched. The closer the saddle then comes the better, if neither the weight of the rider nor settling of the pannel can possibly injure the withers or chine. Before mounting, the rider should examine whether the saddle, girth, straps, bits, bridle, &c., are all good and well fixed.

When the saddle is on the horse, the lowest part of the seat should rather be behind its centre, as it is there that the weight of the body should fall, and by that means the thighs can keep their proper position. The best test of the adaptation of the seat is, when the rider, without stirrups or effort, easily falls into his proper place in the saddle.

Stirrups should not be used until the pupil is capable of riding without them. Their proper length is when the upper edge of the horizontal bar reaches a finger's breadth below the inner ankle-bone. When the feet are in the stirrups, the heels should be about two inches lower than the toes. No more than the natural weight of the limbs should be thrown upon them. It is by an accurate position, and an easy play of the ankle and instep, that the stirrup is retained, so as to slip neither forward nor backward, even if the toe be raised for a moment.

The position on horseback with stirrups differs from that without them only in this, that the thigh being, by the stirrup, relieved from the weight of the leg and foot, the knee is slightly bent, and rather before the lines which these form in the position without stirrups. In hussar riding, hunting, &c., the breadth of four fingers should intervene between the fork and the saddle when the rider stands up.

Spurs should never be used but by an accomplished rider. When it is necessary to employ them, they should be applied a few inches behind the girth, as low as possible, and with the lightest touch capable of producing the effect.

As to the bridle, in order to give the greatest possible ease to the snaffle, a large and polished bit is necessary. Most bits are too small and long, bend back over the bars of the horse's jaw, work like pincers, and cut his mouth.

To give the greatest degree of severity, the bit, while hot, is twisted into a spiral form, so as to present to the jaw a rough and sharp surface, capable of pressing the bars or lips with greater or less severity. The degree of punishment which this bit is capable of inflicting are generally sufficient for all the purposes of correction. It is therefore best to ride with a snaffle, and to use a curb only occasionally when absolutely necessary. In all cases, the rider should observe that the horse is furnished with a bit proper for him. If too light, it may have the effect already described. If too heavy, it may incline him to carry the head low, or to rest upon the hand, which jockeys call "making use of a fifth leg." The simplest and most useful of the *curb* kind is the Weymouth bit, which consists of a strong plain mouth-piece of uniform thickness, without any upset, but merely a curve forwards, to give ease to the tongue.

The centre of the reins should be accurately marked; and, when both reins are held in one hand, and the near rein has to pass under the little finger, and over the fore-finger, on the outside of the off-rein, the latter should be held about half an inch shorter, and the centre should be brought proportionally towards the left. In adjusting the bridle on the horse's head, the head-stall, parallel to and above the cheek-bone, must have its length so regulated as to permit the mouth-piece of the curb to rest on the bars, an inch above the lower tushes in horses, and about two inches above the corner teeth in mares, which have no tushes. The nose-band, lying under the snaffle headstall, must be buckled so loosely that a finger can pass freely under it and over the horse's nose. The bit of the snaffle must be higher, but not so much so as to wrinkle the corner of the mouth. The throat-lash must be buckled rather loose. The mane is usually cut close under the headstall; the finger clears any part of the foretop interfering with it; and the remainder, when combed smooth, is put either over or under the front.

If the rider uses a curb he should make it a rule to hook on the chain himself; for the quietest horse may bring his rider into danger, if the curb hurt him. The curb-chain must pass under the snaffle. The rider should, therefore, put his right hand under the snaffle reins to take hold of the curb-chain, and introducing two fingers of his left within the cheek of the bit, and aiding these with his thumb, take hold of the curb hook. The end links of the curb-chain being in his right hand, he should turn the chain to the right and under, or as he would a screw, till every link lies flat and smooth, and then, without losing a half turn, put that link on the hook which appears to be neither tight nor slack. The finger should pass between the horse's jaw

14

and curb, which in this case hangs down upon his under lip. It is necessary also to see how it operates. If the branch has liberty to move forty-five degrees, or to a right angle, it is the degree which is in general best. If, however, one link of the chain confine it to thirty-five degrees, and if one link lower give it fifty-five degrees, then the manner of the horse's carrying his head must determine which is most proper: if the horse naturally carry his nose high, the branch may have fifty-five; if he bring his nose in, he should have thirty-five degrees. If there be a chain-strap, it must be placed so high on the branch, that when passed passed through the ring in the curb-chin, it may be buckled tight enough to prevent the horse lodging the branch on his teeth.

When a horse's head is steady, when he is light in hand, can obey its motions with ease, and stop readily, the bit is properly adjusted. On the contrary, if he open his mouth as if gagged, writhe his jaws, draw his tongue above the mouth-piece, or thrust it out sidewise; if he fear the impression of the bit, have no appuy, toss his head up and down, carry it low, and endeavor to force the hand, or refuse to go forward, or run backward, the bit is not properly adjusted.

MOUNTING AND DISMOUNTING.

In mounting, the rider,—presenting himself rather before the horse's shoulder, with his left breast towards that shoulder, and with his whip or switch in his left hand,—takes, with the right hand, the snaffle reins in the centre; introduces the little finger of the left hand between them from before, the back of that hand being towards the horse's head;—places the left hand below the right on the neck of the horse, about twelve inches from the saddle;—

Plate.XXVI.

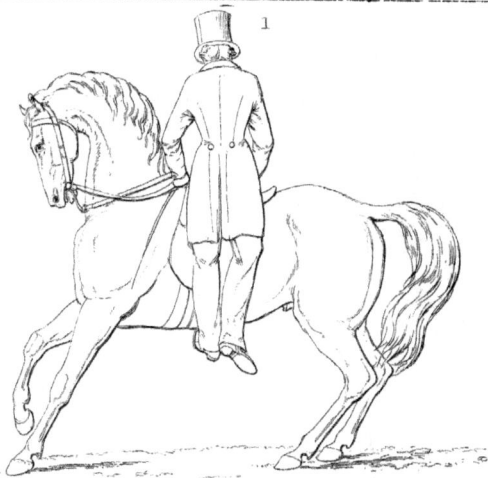

Second View of Mounting.

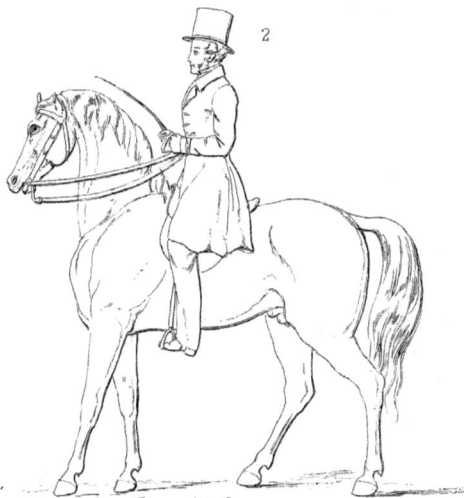

The Seat

draws with the right hand the reins through the left, and shortens them, till the left has a light and equal feeling of both reins on the horse's mouth;—throws, with the right hand, the reins to the off side;—takes, with the same hand, a lock of the mane, brings it through the left hand, and turns it round the left thumb:—and closes the left hand firmly on the mane and reins.

The right hand, after quitting the mane, lays hold of the left stirrup, the fingers being behind, and the thumb in front of it; the left foot is raised and put into the stirrup as far as the ball of it, (Pl. XXXV. fig. 2,) the right foot is then moved until the rider's face is turned to the side of the horse, and looking across the saddle; while the right hand is placed on the cantle, the left knee against the saddle on the surcingle, with the left heel drawn back, to avoid touching the horse's side with the toe; by a spring of the right foot from the instep, not by any pull with the right hand, the rider raises himself in the stirrup, the knees firm against the saddle, the heels together, but drawn back a little, and the body erect, and partially supported by the right hand, (Pl. XXXVI. fig. 1,) the right hand moves from the cantle to the pommel, and supports the body; the right leg at the same time passes clearly over the horse's quarters to the off side; the right knee closes on the saddle; the body comes gently into it; the left hand quits the mane, and the right the pommel.

The left, or bridle hand, with the wrist rounded outwards, is placed opposite the centre of the body, and at three inches' distance from it; the right hand is dropped by the side of the thigh; the stirrup is taken instantly with the right foot, without the help of hand or eye; the clothes are adjusted; and the whip is exchanged from the left hand to the right, being held with the lash upwards, but inclining a little towards the left ear of the horse, and never leaving the right hand, except while mounting or dismounting,—(Plate XXXVI. fig. 2.)

The horse is to be accustomed to stand till the rider request him to move. The habit of unsteadiness is acquired from grooms, who, on going out to water and exercise, throw themselves over a horse from some elevation, and give a kick to the animal even before being fairly upon it. If a groom attend at mounting, he ought not to be suffered to touch the reins, but only that part of the bridle which comes down the cheek.

In dismounting, the whip is to be returned into the left hand; the right hand takes hold of the rein above the left; the right foot quits the stirrup; the left hand slides forward on the rein, to about twelve inches from the saddle, feeling the horse's mouth very lightly; the right hand, dropping the reins to the off side, takes a lock of the mane, brings it through the left, and twists it round the left thumb; the fingers of the left hand close on it; the right hand is placed on the pommel; the body being kept erect. The body is supported with the right hand and left foot; the right leg is, without touching the horse's hind-quarters or the saddle, brought gently to the near side, with the heels close, care being taken not to bend the right knee, lest the spur should touch the horse; the right hand passes at the same time to the cantle, to preserve the balance, as in the act of mounting; the body is gently lowered until the right toe touches the ground; resting on the right foot, the left stirrup is quitted, and the left foot placed in line with the horse's hoofs; the hands remaining as in the former motion. Both hands then quit their holds of the mane and cantle; and the right hand lays hold of the snaffle rein near the ring of the bit.

In mounting without stirrups,—after taking up the reins, instead of seizing the mane, the rider lays hold of the pommel and cantle, and, by a spring of both legs from the insteps, raises the body to the centre of the saddle. By a second spring of both arms, the right leg is carried over the horse, and the rider enters his proper seat by closing the knees on the saddle, and sliding gently into it.

In dismounting without stirrups, on either side of the horse, the rider throws the weight of the body on the hands placed on the pommel, and, by a spring, raises the body out of the saddle, before the leg is brought over the horse.

THE SEAT.

The seat must be understood in an extended sense as the disposition of the various parts of the body, in conformity with the action of the horse; and its effect is the rider's being firm in the saddle, when he might be otherwise thrown forward over the horse's head, or backward over his tail.

The fundamental seat is that intermediate one of which all others are modifications, and in which the rider sits when the horse is going straight forward, without any bend in his position. In describing this, it is first necessary to consider the rider's relation to the horse. He must sit on that part of the animal's body which, as he springs in his paces, is the centre of motion; from which, of course, any weight would be most difficultly shaken. The place of this seat is that part of the saddle into which the rider's body would naturally slide were he to ride without stirrups. This seat is to be preserved only by a proper balance of his body, and its adaptation to even the most

violent counteractions of the horse. Turf jockeys necessarily sit further back, that they may employ the pulls.

It is necessary to consider the horseman in various parts,
and to explain their different functions: 1st, the lower
part, as being here the principal one, namely, the thighs,
with the legs as dependent on them; 2dly, the upper part,
namely, the body, with the arms dependent on it. The
thighs, from the fork to the knees, are commonly called
the immovable parts, and upon them the whole attitude
depends. They must not wriggle or roll, so as either to
disturb the horse, or render the seat loose; but they may
be relaxed when the horse hesitates to advance. The legs
occasionally strengthen the hold of the thighs by a grasp
with the calves; and they likewise aid, support, and chas-
tise the horse. The body, from the fork upwards, must
always be in a situation to take the corresponding motion,
and preserve the balance. The position of the arms is
dependent on that of the body, but they also exercise new
functions.

As a good seat is the basis of all excellence in riding,
we shall consider these parts in detail.

In relation to the thighs, the rider, sitting in the middle
of the saddle, must rest chiefly upon their division, vulgarly
called the fork, and very slightly upon the hips. The
thighs, turned inward, must rest flat upon the sides of the
saddle, without grasping; for the rider's weight gives
sufficient hold, and the pressure of the thighs on the saddle
would only lift him above it. The knees must be stretched
down and kept back, so as to place the thighs several
degrees short of a perpendicular; but no gripe must be
made with them, unless there be danger of losing all other
hold. If the thighs are upon their inner or flat side in
the saddle, both the legs and the feet will be turned as

they ought to be. Thus turned, they must be on a line parallel to that of the rider's body, and hang near the horse's sides, but must not touch; yet they may give an additional hold to the seat, when necessary, and the calves must act in support of the aids of the hands. The heels are to be sunk, and the toes to be raised, and as near the horse as the heels, which prevents the heel touching the horse.

As to the body.—The head must be firm, yet free. The shoulders thrown back, and kept square, so that no pull of the bridle may bring them forward. The chest must be advanced, and the small of the back bent a little forward.

The upper parts of the arms must hang perpendicularly from the shoulders, the lower parts at right angles with the upper, so as to form a horizontal line from the elbow to the little finger. The elbows must be lightly closed to the hips, and, without stiffness, kept steady, or they destroy the hand. The wrist must be rounded a little outwards. The hands should be about three inches from the body, and from the pommel of the saddle, and from four to six inches apart; the thumbs and knuckles pointing towards each other, and the finger nails towards the body.*

When the rider is in the proper position on horseback without stirrups, his nose, breast, knee, and instep are nearly in a line; and, with stirrups, his nose, breast, knee, and toe are in a line. (Pl. XXXVI.) The man and the horse throughout are to be of a piece. When the horse is at liberty, or disunited, as it is termed, the rider sits at his ease; and as he collects and unites his horse, so he collects and unites himself. There must, however, be no

* When in motion round the manege, or the circle, the inward hand, or that towards which we turn, is to be a little lower than the outward one.

stiffness of manner, more than in sitting on a chair; for it
is ease and elegance which distinguish the gentleman.

THE BALANCE.

The balance in riding preserves the body from that inclination to one side or the other which even the ordinary
paces of the horse, in the trot or gallop, would otherwise
occasion.   It accompanies and corresponds with every
motion of the animal, without any employment of strength,
and consequently, the rider sits so firmly that nothing can
move his seat.   His skill consists essentially in balancing
himself on the horse in such a manner as not to fetter the
animal's movements.   To illustrate this, if the horse work
straight and upright on his legs, the body must be in the
same upright direction : as the horse moves into a trot, the
body must be inclined a little more back; in the gallop,
also in leaping, or in any violent movements, the body must
chiefly be kept back ; and, when the horse bends and leans,
as he does when on a circle, or trotting briskly round a
corner, the body must lean similarly, or the balance will
be lost.   Throughout the whole, the figure must be pliant
to every action of the horse; for the balance can be maintained only by as many different positions as he is capable
of working in.

To help his balance, the rider must never take the
slightest assistance from the reins.   Whatever the position
of the body, the hand must be fixed, and the reins of such
a length as to feel and support the horse, but never to hold
on.   To acquire the balance, the practice on circles, or the
longe, is useful; working equally to both hands, and not
using stirrups till the pupil has acquired the balance
without them.   Experience proves that the body, if in the

manege seat and fundamental position, almost involuntarily takes the corresponding motion, whether the horse stumbles, rears, springs forward, or kicks.

THE REIN-HOLD.

There are various methods of holding the reins, according to the style of riding, the design of the rider, and the propensities of horses.

In holding the snaffle-reins separately, one rein passes into each hand, between the third and fourth fingers, and out of it over the fore-finger, where it is held down by the thumb —(Plate XXXVII. fig. 1.) When afterwards further advanced, the reins are held in the left hand, as at first taken up; the left rein passing under the little finger, and the right under the third finger, both lying smooth through the hand, the superfluous rein hanging over the first joint of the fore-finger, and the thumb being placed upon it.*— (Plate XXXVII. fig. 2.)

Riders should not throw their right shoulders back, as they are apt to do, when they first take the reins in one hand. The right arm should hang by the side, with the hand by the side of the thigh; or, if holding the whip, it may be kept a little lower than the left, in order not to obstruct the operation of the bridle.

We have already said, that we think it best to ride with the snaffle alone, and use the curb only occasionally. In this case, the curb reins may have a slide upon them, and hang on the pommel of the saddle, or the horse's neck.

* Sometimes, however, the right rein is made to enter the hand from above over the fore-finger, and crosses the left rein in the palm, where the fingers close upon them, a loop or bow being formed of the residue between the hand and the body, whence it hangs down.—(Plate XXXVII. fig. 3.)

When the rider, however, holds the curb as well as the snaffle, having both, as is most usual, in the left hand,— while the curb reins are placed as above described of the snaffle reins, the snaffle reins are placed within them ; that is, the left snaffle rein enters under the second, and the right under the first finger, and both pass up through the hand, and out of it, over the fore-finger, precisely as do the curb reins, except that they lie at first above, then within, and lastly, under them.—(Plate XXXVII. fig. 4.)

Shifting the reins should be done expertly, without stopping the horse, altering the pace, breaking the time, or looking to the hands. When the snaffle reins are held in one hand, the method of shifting from the left hand is as follows :—Turn the thumbs towards each other; carry the right hand over the left; in place of the little finger of the left hand, put the fore-finger of the right hand downwards between the reins ; lay the reins smoothly down through the right hand, and place the thumb upon the left rein between the first and second joint of the fore-finger.— (Plate XXXVII. fig. 5.) To shift them again into the left hand, it is only necessary to carry the left hand over the right ; to put the little finger of the left hand downwards between the right and left reins; to place them smoothly upwards through the hand, and to let the ends hang over the fore-finger, as at first.—(Plate XXXVII. fig. 6.)

When both curb and snaffle reins are held in the usual method, we shift them into the right hand in a similar manner, by turning the thumbs towards each other; carrying the right hand over the left; putting the fore-finger of the right hand into the place of the little finger of the left; the second finger of the right into the place of the third finger of the left; and the third finger of the right into the place of the second finger of the left; and laying the reins

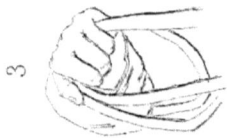

3

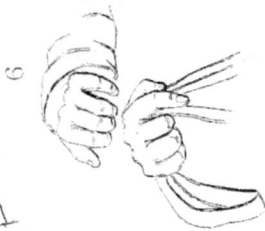

6

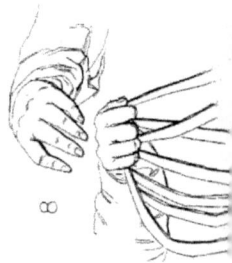

7

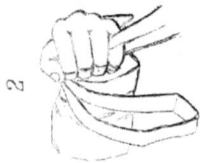

2

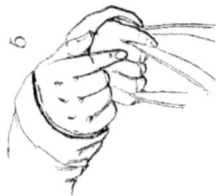

4

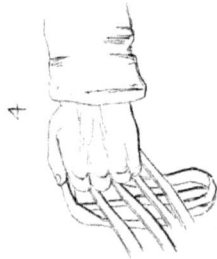

5

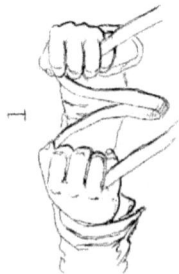

1

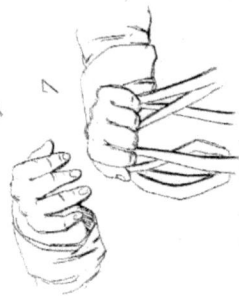

9

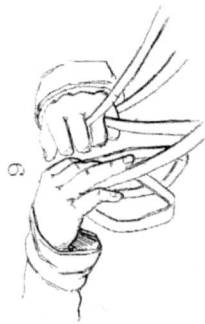

8

smoothly down through the right hand.—(Plate XXXVII.
fig. 7.) When we shift the reins again to the left hand, we
put the fingers of the left hand into the places we took them
from, and turn the reins smoothly upward through the
hand, and over the fore-finger.—(Plate XXXVII. fig. 8.)

Separating the reins is sometimes necessary. When a
horse refuses obedience to one hand, we use two. It is
seldom, however, necessary to take more than one rein in
the right hand ; and this is the right rein of the snaffle
only. For this purpose, the rider turns the back of his
right hand upwards, puts the first three fingers over the
snaffle rein, receives it between his little and third fingers,
lets the superfluous end hang over the fore-finger, with the
thumb upwards, as he does the bridle hand. (Plate
XXXVII. fig. 9.)

Adjusting the reins is shortening or lengthening them,
wholly or partially, as occasion may require. To adjust
the whole, we take the superfluous reins that hang over the
fore-finger of the left hand into the right, so that with that
hand we support the horse, and feel every step he takes ;
and we then open the fingers of the left hand so as to slip
it up and down the reins smoothly and freely, and thereby
adjust them to our pleasure.

To shorten the curb rein, and lengthen the snaffle, we
take in the right hand the centre of the curb rein, that
hangs over the fore-finger, slip the whole of the reins too
long, pass the left hand down them, and feel with the
fingers whether both the curb reins are of equal length,
before we grasp with the left hand, or quit with the right.
Similarly, we shorten the snaffle, and lengthen the curb,
by taking in the right hand the centre of the snaffle that
hangs over the fore-finger, and proceeding in the same way.

When any single rein wants shortening, we apply the

right hand to that part which hangs over the fore-finger, and draw it tighter. When the reins are separate, or occupy both hands, and want adjusting, we bring the hands together to assist each other; remembering that the inner hand, or that which supports the attitude the horse works in, is not to depart from its situation, so as to occasion any disorder, but that the outer hand is to be brought to the inner, for the purpose of adjusting them.

THE CORRESPONDENCE.

To have a correct notion of the manner in which the hand operates on the horse's mouth, it must be understood that the reins, being held as described, are collected to such definite length, that bracing the muscles of the hand would rein the horse back, and easing them permit him freely to advance; the hand, for preserving a medium effect on the mouth, being only half shut, and the knuckles near the wrist nearly open. The hand, then, being connected to the reins, the reins to the bit, the bit operating in the curb on the bars, and in the snaffle on the lips, the rider cannot move the hand, and scarcely even a finger, without the horse's mouth being more or less affected. This is called the CORRESPONDENCE.

If, moreover, the hand be held steady, as the horse advances in the trot, the fingers will feel, by the contraction of the reins, a slight tug, occasioned by the cadence of every step; and this tug, by means of the correspondence, is reciprocally felt in the horses mouth. This is called the APPUY.

While this relation is preserved between the hand and mouth, the horse is in perfect obedience to the rider, and the hand directs him, in any position or action, with such ease, that the horse seems to work by the will of the rider rather than by the power of his hand. This is called the SUPPORT.

Now, the correspondence or effective communication between the hand and mouth,—the appuy, or strength of the operation in the mouth,—the support, or aid, the hand gives in the position or action,—are always maintained in the manège and all united paces. Without these, a horse is under no immediate control, as in the extended gallop, or at full speed, where it may require a hundred yards to pull before we can stop him.

THE ACTION.

The degree of correspondence, appuy, and support, depends, in horses otherwise similar, on the relative situation of the hand. The act of raising the rider's hand increases his power; and this, raising the horse's head, diminishes his power. The depressing of the rider's hand, on the contrary, diminishes his power; and this, depressing the horse's head, increases his power. On these depend the unitedness or disunitedness in the action of the horse.

A writer on this subject (Beranger, we believe,) gives the following useful illustration :—" If a garter were placed across the pupil's forehead, and a person behind him held the two ends in a horizontal direction, the pupil, if he stood quite upright, could not pull at the person's hand, nor endure the person's hand to pull at him, without falling or running backwards." This is the situation of a horse when united.

Accordingly, when the pupil felt the hand severe, or expected it to pull, he would guard against it by bending the body, projecting the head, and planting one foot behind. This is the situation of a horse when disunited, or defending himself against the heaviness of the hand.

15

Hence the perpetual pull of a timid rider, or a heavy insensible hand, cannot keep a horse united, because the horse cannot then bear its severity. Thus heavy hands make hard-mouthed horses; and hence it is in this condition that we generally find horses, for the best broke become so, if ridden a few times by an ignorant horseman. In such cases, the horse makes the rider support the weight both of his head and neck, or goes on his shoulders, and is apt to stumble.

If, then, the appuy be heavy, from the head being carried too low, and the horse not sufficiently united, the rider must raise the hand, and let the fingers, by moving, rather invite than compel the head, or more properly the neck, to rise, for the object is to bring in the head by raising the neck, the legs at the same time pressing the haunches under. By these means, the horse will be united, and the appuy will be lightened. Should the hand, however, be too confining to the horse when united, he may become so balanced on his haunches that he can neither disunite himself nor advance one step; and, should the rider then press him without yielding or dropping the hand, he would compel him to rear.

Such are the two extremes, where the horse is disunited, and where he is too much united. The intermediate effect of the hand and heel must be acquired by practice.

THE HAND.

To a masterly hand, firmness, gentleness, and lightness, are very properly described as being essentially necessary.

Firmness of the hand does not, however, do more than correspond exactly with the feeling in the horse's mouth, unless the horse attempts to get the ascendency, to abandon that delicate correspondence producing the appuy, and keeping him under the strictest obedience, and to make a dull or insensible pull on the hand. To frustrate these attemps, the hand is kept firm, and the fingers braced; and, should the horse plant his head low to endure this, the fingers are moved, the reins shaken, &c., to raise the head and divert him from his purpose; or, if this be unavailing, the hand is yielded that the reins may become slack, and a snatch is given in an upward direction, which will not only make him raise his head, but will deter him from putting it down again.

Gentleness of the hand relaxes a little of its firmness, and mitigates the feeling between the hand and the horse's mouth, without passing, however, from one extreme to another. Lightness of the hand lessens still more the feeling between the rider's hand and the horses mouth, and consists in a slight alternate feeling and easing of the bridle, regulated by the motion of the horse: for, if the appuy were always in the same degree, it would heat the mouth, dull the feeling, and render the horse's bars callous. The rider must also distinguish whether the horse wishes to disengage himself from restriction, or wants a momentary liberty to cough, to move if cramped, to dislodge a fly, &c.

The curb, if used, requires always a light hand to manage it; and the horse should never be put to do any thing in a curb at which he is not perfectly ready. The curb is adapted for acting in a direct line only: the snaffle should be used in all other cases. Still, as to all these qualities, the transitions must be gradual. Were the rider, passing over that degree of restraint which is derived from the easy or gentle hand, to go at once from a firm to a slack one, he would deprive his horse of the support he trusted to, and precipitate him on his shoulders. On the contrary, were he to pass from the slack to the tight rein all at once, he would give a violent shock to the horse's mouth.

All the operations of the hand, then, should be firm, gentle, and light; and in these, the fingers and wrist alone must act. Certain liberties called descents of the hand, are also taken with well-bred horses. These are made three different ways :—by advancing the arm a little, but not the shoulder, still keeping the usual length of rein, or by dropping the knuckles directly and at once upon the horse's neck ;—by taking the reins in the right hand, about four fingers' breadth above the left, and letting them slide through the left, dropping the right hand at the same time upon the horse's neck ;—and by taking the end of the reins in the right hand, quitting them entirely with the left, and letting the end of them fall upon the horse's neck. These graceful freedoms must never be used but with great caution, when the horse is quite together, and in hand; and the rider, by throwing back his body, must counterbalance the weight of the horse upon his haunches.

There are still minuter rules belonging to this head; for instance, both snaffle reins being in one hand, and that in the first position,—if we open the first and second fingers, we slacken the right rein ;—if we open the little finger, we slacken the left rein ;—if we shut the hand entirely, and immediately open it again, we lessen the tension of both reins. By these methods, we may relieve and freshen the two bars in which the feeling and appuy resides. So also in the second descent of the hand. While the right hand holds the reins, we may slide the left hand up and down these in that degree of appuy which belongs to the easy and slack hand : during which the horse will endeavor to preserve that mutual sensation between the mouth and the hand, which makes him submit with pleasure to constraint. By this play of the rein and movement of the bit to avoid pressure in one continued way, the horse's head is kept high, and his neck and crest are raised.

THE GUIDANCE OR AIDS.

The modes of guiding the horse are called aids, because they not only direct, but assist him to execute. They also check him in acting contrarily. These aids are certain positions of the hand, body, legs, and sometimes of the switch or whip. The hand is so far the principal of these, that the others are sometimes called accompaniments, as only giving power and efficacy to the hand.

Aids of the Hand.

A horse can move four different ways—forward, to the right, to the left, and backward; but he cannot perform these motions unless the hand of the rider makes four corresponding motions. There are accordingly five different positions for the hand, including the general one from which the other four proceed.

The five Positions when one Rein is held in each Hand.

In the first position, the reins pass up between the third and fourth fingers of each hand, their ends are thrown over the fore-fingers, the thumbs are closed on them, and the fingers are shut :—the hands being held as already described in treating of the seat. The second position consists of a slight relaxation of the preceding, and permits the horse to advance. The third position shortens the right rein rather upward, and turns the horse to the right. The fourth position shortens the left rein rather upward, and turns the horse to the left; and the fifth position shortens both reins, and stops or reins the horse backwards.

The five positions when the Reins are held in one Hand.

The aids of the hand, as forming these positions, when

the reins are held in one hand, may be very simply given by a little extending, or bending the wrist, to make the horse advance, or go backward,—and by slightly carrying the hand to the right or to the left, and in both cases rather upward, to make the horse turn in these directions.

The Twistings of the Bridle Hand.

Several modifications of the rules already given occur. We do not, however, approve of these positions, as they, in a great measure, reverse and destroy the natural aids of the hand, by leaving the right rein slack in the turn to the right, and the left rein slack in the turn to the left. Indeed, they could not possibly be obeyed by the horse, were it not that, on this point, he seems to have more understanding than his rider, and draws his conclusions as to the latter's intentions, not from the inconsistent action of his hand, but from the more natural accompanying aids of his body and legs. Fortunately, however, these twistings of the bridle hand, though always taught, are, we believe, rarely practised.

We give these positions here, only in compliance with custom.

In the first position the under surface of the fore-arm and hand forms a horizontal line from the elbow to the joint of the little finger; the elbow is lightly closed to the hips; the wrist is rounded; the knuckles are kept directly above the neck of the horse, the hand being at three inches from the body, and as much from the pommel of the saddle; the nails are turned towards the body, the little finger being nearer to it than the others; the reins, in entering the hand, are separated by the little finger; and the thumb is placed flat upon them as they pass out over the fore-finger.

In the second position the hand is yielded to the horse

by turning the nails downward, so as to carry the thumb nearer the body, and the little finger further from it, yet somewhat obliquely, for the thumb passes nearly into the place where the knuckles were in the first position, the nails being now directly above the horse's neck. This permits the horse to advance.

In the third position the hand, leaving the first, is turned upside down, so that the thumb is carried out to the left, and the little finger brought into the right. This carries the operation of the reins nearly three inches more to the right, by which the left reins press the neck, the right reins are slack, and the horse is turned to the right.

In the fourth position the hand, leaving the first, the back is turned upward, so that the little finger is carried out to the left, and the thumb brought in to the right. This carries the operation of the reins to the left, by which the right reins press the neck, the left reins are slack, and the horse is turned to the left.

In the fifth position, quitting the first, the wrist is rounded, the nails turned upwards, and the knuckles towards the horse's neck. This stops him, or compels him to go backward.

These aids, however, when the reins are held in one hand, are not so effective as those where the reins are separate.

Aids of the Body.

To aid the second position of the hand, and cause the horse to advance, the body may be thrown a little forward, but not so as to press heavily on his fore-parts. To aid the third and fourth positions of the hand, a mere turn of the body is sufficient. Thus, in entering an angle, it is only necessary to turn the body imperceptibly toward the corner, just as if the rider intended to go into it himself; his body then turning to the right or left, his hand must necessarily turn likewise, and the leg of the side on which he turns will infallibly press against the horse, and aid him. In coming out of a corner, it is only necessary to turn the body again, the hand will follow it, and the other leg, approaching the horse, will put his croupe into the corner, in such a manner that it will follow the shoulders, and be upon the same line. The same motion of the body is likewise necessary to turn entirely to the right or left. To aid the fifth position of the hand, and make the horse go backward, the body must be thrown gently back, and the hand will go with it.

Aids of the Legs.

To aid the second position of the hand, and make the horse advance, the legs must be closed. Even when a horse stands still, the legs held near him will keep him on the watch, and with the slightest upward motion of the bridle, he will raise his head and show his forehead to advantage. To aid the third position of the hand, and turn to the right, the right leg must determine the croupe to the left, and facilitate the action of the shoulder, which the hand had turned to the right. To aid the fourth position of the hand, and turn to the left, the left leg must determine the croupe to the right. In making a change to the right, the left leg confines the croupe, so that it must follow the shoulders.— In changing again to the left, the right leg acts similarly. To aid the fifth position of the hand, and stop the horse, while he is held in, the legs must be gently brought to the sides.

The aids of the legs have their degrees progressively increasing, thus :—the leg being brought nearer the side is the lightest; placing the leg further back, with the toe turned out, is the next; a touch with the calf of the leg, is the third; a stroke with it, having the toe kept up firmly, that the muscles of the leg may be hard, is the fourth; and the strongest is the scratch, which, when the legs are laid on hard without effect, is given by dropping the toe, when, if the spur be properly placed, the rowel will scratch the horse's side, and this is succeeded by giving the spur sharply. Aids with the whip are also used to give greater effect to the heel. These are gentle taps on the hind quarters, and sometimes on the shoulders. When given on the near side, the hand is either applied behind the back, with the whip held by the fingers like a pen, the lash being downwards, or across the bridle-hand before, the whip being help with the lash upwards.

ANIMATIONS, SOOTHINGS, AND CORRECTIONS.

Animations proceed from the hand, the leg, the whip, or the tongue; those of the hand and of the legs have been described among the aids. Animations of the whip are mild taps to quicken the horse, or, if the lash is upwards, switching it in the air. Those of the leg and whip threaten punishment; and accordingly, with sluggish horses, both may be necessary. The animation of the tongue is produced by placing the tongue flat against the roof of the mouth, and suddenly displacing the posterior part of it by drawing the air laterally between it and the palate. This noise is animating to the horse; but, if too much continued, or too frequent, its effect is destroyed.

Soothings are the reverse of animations, and are used to dispel the fears of horses, and to give them confidence. The voice soothes by soft and mild tones; the hand, by gentle patting, or stroking; the body and legs, by relinquishing all unnecessary firmness, and sitting easy. A

horseman should have perfect command of his temper, as
well as invincible patience and perseverance, to make the
horse comprehend and perform. He must demand but
little the first time; he will be more readily obeyed the
next; and he may increase his demands as the horse improves in habit and temper.

Corrections are given either with the spurs or switch, or
by keeping the horse in a greater degree of subjection.
In these a good horseman endeavors rather to work upon
the mind than the body of the horse. The corrections
which render a horse most obedient, and yet dishearten
him least, are not severe, but rather oppose him by restraint, and make him do directly the contrary. If, for
example, he do not go off readily, or if he be sluggish,
make him go sidewise, sometimes to one hand, sometimes
the other, then drive him forward. If he go forward too
fast, moderate the aids, and make him go backward more
or less according to his conduct. If he be disorderly and
turbulent, walk him straight forward, with head in and
croupe out.

When correction is given with the whip, it should be
with strength; the lash being upwards, the arm lifted
high, and the whip applied behind the girths round the
belly: or it may be given forward, over the shoulders,
between the fore-legs. Should the horse kick at the application of the whip to his flank or quarter, the rider must
instantly apply it smartly, and must repeat it more sharply,
should he kick at that. By this he may be made sensible
of his fault.

To give a horse both spurs properly, the rider must
change the posture of his legs, and, bending his knee,
strike him with them at once, quickly and firmly. Some
horses disregard the whip, but fly at the spurs; others

disregard the spurs, and are terrified at the whip; the rider consequently will apply that which is most likely to produce the desired effect. When, however, the whip or spurs are applied two or three times sharply to restive horses without effect, the rider must desist and try other methods.

THE WALK.

The rider should not suffer his horse to move till his clothes are adjusted, and whip shifted, when, collecting his reins, and taking one in his right hand, he must close his legs, to induce the horse to move slowly forward in the walk. If he wish to increase the pace, the pressure of the knees must be increased. When the horse moves, the legs must resume their former position,—the hands remain perfectly steady,—and the body yield to the movement.

As to character, the walk is the pace performed with the least exertion; only one leg at a time being off the ground, and three on. In this pace, accordingly, four distinct beats are marked, as each foot comes to the ground in the following order:—first the off fore foot, next the near hind foot, then the near fore foot, and lastly, the off hind foot.*

The perfection of the walk consists in its being an animated quick step, measuring exact distances, and marking a regular time, by putting the feet flat to the ground. Its excellence depends on that uniting of the horse which supports his head and raises his feet, without shortening or retarding the step; and that animation

---

* The amble may perhaps be considered as a natural pace, as most foals, following their dams, amble more or less to keep up with them. The difference between the walk and the amble is, that two legs of a side are raised in the latter at the same instant.

which quickens the step and sharpens the beats without altering the time or the action.

In performance, if the rider do not support the horse sufficiently, his head will be low; and his walk slovenly: if he support him too much, he will shorten his step so that he cannot walk freely. If the rider do not animate him, he will not exert himself: if he animate him too much, he will trot. If the horse trot when the rider designs him to walk, he will find either his hand or the degree of animation communicated by the whip, tongue, legs, or bracing of the body, too high, and this he must instantly modify, as well as check the horse. (Plate XXXVIII. fig. 1.)

Turns in the Walk.

Turns in general should be made slowly; and all the aids should combine in producing them.

In performance, the hand to which we turn, or inner hand, is to be a little below the outer one, and the inner rein held with double the force of the outer one, which is to be exerted by the little finger pulling gently upwards and towards the body, while the outer hand retains a steady hold of the outer rein. At the same time, the legs, by a slight pressure with the calves, must support the horse, keep him up to the bridle, make him bring his haunches under him, and obey the leading rein. The pressure of the inward leg alone would make him throw his haunches too much outwards. All this is to be done in proportion to the effect meant to be produced; and great precision and delicacy are required in the execution.

Wheels may also be briefly noticed here. A horse may wheel or turn on his own ground, on three pivots,—on his centre, on his fore feet, and on his hind feet. In all these,

Plate XXXVIII

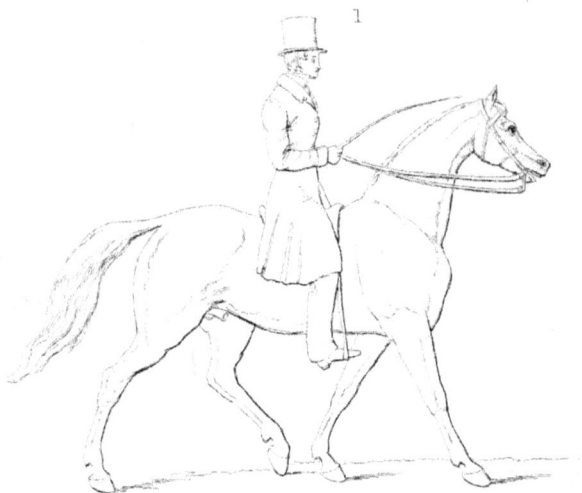

The Walk

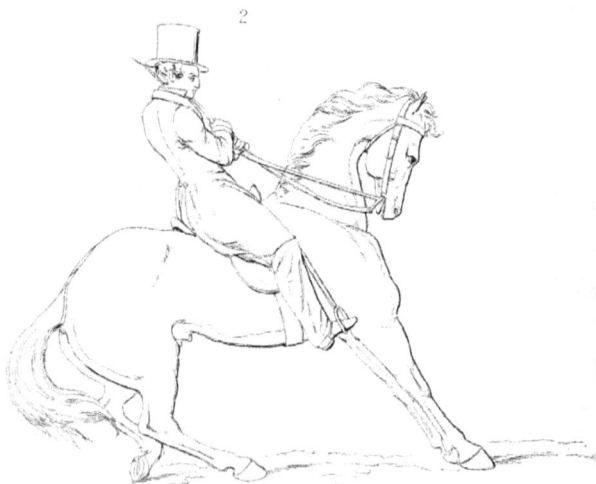

The Stop

the hand directs all before the horseman, and the heel all
behind him. In wheeling on centres, the hand and heel
operate together—the hand leading the shoulder round—
the leg directing the croupe, by which means, in going
about, the fore feet describe one half circle, and the hind
feet another. Here the aids of the hand, body, and legs,
must exactly correspond; and the degree of appuy must
be merely such as will carry its aid into effect; for, if the
appuy is too weak, the horse will advance over his ground,
and if too strong, he will retire from it.

.On terminating the wheel or quarter circle, the about
or half circle, or the about and about, or whole circle, the
hand, the body, and leg, must instantly resume their proper position. The wheel on the fore, and that on the hind
feet, are still more rarely of use in common practice.

Stops in the Walk.

Horses and horsemen generally stop by a gradual cessation of action, in a time and distance which depend on
circumstances. As to character, however, the stop, when
properly performed, is an instant cessation of advance,
without any previous indication.

When the stop is properly performed, it shows the great
superiority of the rider's hand over the horse. It confirms
him in obedience, unites him, supples the haunches, and
bends the houghs. Much mischief, however, may occur
from a too frequent or injudicious practice of it. The
perfection of the stop consists in the action ceasing at the
finish of a cadence, without breaking the previous time;
and in the horse being so balanced on his haunches, and
so animated, that, with liberty given, he can advance with
the same rapidity as before.

In performance, the time to be seized is when the first
16

part of the cadence is coming to the ground; so that its finish completes the stop. If this is not done, the cadence will be broken, and the stop rendered irregular. At such a moment, the stop is performed by the rider bracing his arms to his body, holding both reins equally and firmly, drawing the fingers towards the body, closing for an instant both legs, to press the horse up to the bridle, and throwing the body back, with precisely such strength of all the muscles as is proportioned to the effect; all this being done at the same instant, and making but one motion. If the rider do not close his legs, the horse may not bring his haunches under, the stop will be on the shoulders, and its effect will be destroyed.

If, in stopping, a horse toss up his nose, or force the hand, the bridle hand must be kept low and firm, no liberty must be given, his neck must be pressed with the right hand till he has brought down his nose, and immediately all his bridle may be given him. (Pl. XXXVIII. fig. 2.) If the horse has not readily obeyed, he should be made to go backwards, as a proper punishment for the fault.

Going Backward in the Walk.

The action of the horse when he goes backward is to bend his haunches, to have always one of his hinder legs under his belly, on which to rest and balance himself, and to push his croupe backward. In performance, the horse's head must be steady and right, his body gathered up under him, he must be upon his haunches, and his feet be even. To aid him in this, there should be an equal and steady feeling of both reins; the hand must be held centrically, and kept from rising, with the knuckles a little down, inviting the horse to back; the body bent a little forward, with the belly drawn in, and the legs gently pressing the sides of the horse, in order to keep him up to the bridle, and to prevent him from swerving.

The instant he yields to the hand, the body and hand yield to the horse, that he may recover his balance; and he may then be pressed to back again. If either the deviation of the hand from its centrical situation, or any other cause, make the croupe go off the line in an opposite direction, the heel must support and direct him. Thus, should the croupe traverse to the right, the right leg must direct; and, to assist, the hand must be carried a little to the right; but this must be done with delicacy, lest the croupe be thrown too much to the left. Here the hand and the heel change their functions; the hand compels the action, and the heel directs it.

THE TROT.

As to the character of the trot, when we urge the horse to proceed faster than he can by moving one leg after the other in the walk, we oblige him to take up two at a time in the trot. Here the off fore-foot and the near hind-foot give one beat; and the near fore-foot and the off hind-foot give another; so that there are two legs crosswise off the ground, and two legs on; the beats being sharp and quick, in proportion to the degree of animation and extension.

The perfection of the trot consists in its suppleness, giving the horse a free use of his limbs; in its union, distributing his labor more equally, his fore legs having more to sustain than the hind, especially when he is disunited, or on the shoulders; and in its action, which should be true and equal, the liberty of the fore-quarters not exceeding the hind, nor the hind the fore—the knee being up, the haunches bent, springy, and pliant, the step measuring exact distances, and marking a regular time. In the trot, there is a leading foot, either right or left, by which the coresponding side is little more advanced than the other. This leading with either foot is valuable, as, in horses that have not been thus supplied, if chance or fatigue makes them change their leg for that which they are not accustomed to, the action is stiff, confined, and irregular.

Kinds of Trot.

There are three kinds of trot—the extended, the supple, and the even.

In the extended trot, the horse steps out without retaining himself, being quite straight, and going directly forwards.

In the supple trot, at every motion he bends and plays the joints of his shoulders, knees, and feet.

In the even trot, he makes all his limbs and joints move so equally and exactly, that his limbs never cover more ground one than the other, nor at one time more than at another.

These three kinds of trot depend upon each other. We cannot pass a horse to the supple trot without having first worked him to the extended trot; and we can never arrive at the even and equal trot without having practised the supple. To pass from the extended to the supple trot, the horse must be gently and by degrees held in. When, by exercise, he has attained sufficient suppleness to manage his limbs readily, he must insensibly be held in more and more, till he is led to the equal trot.

The Trot in particular.

In performance the rider must apply, for an instant, both legs to his horse's sides; and at the same time raise the

Plate XXXIX

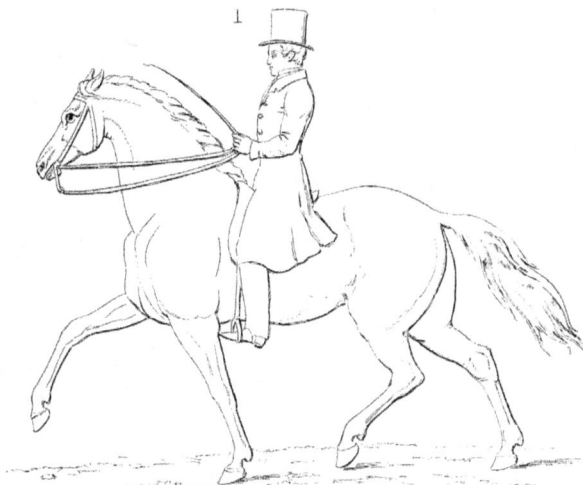

The Trot

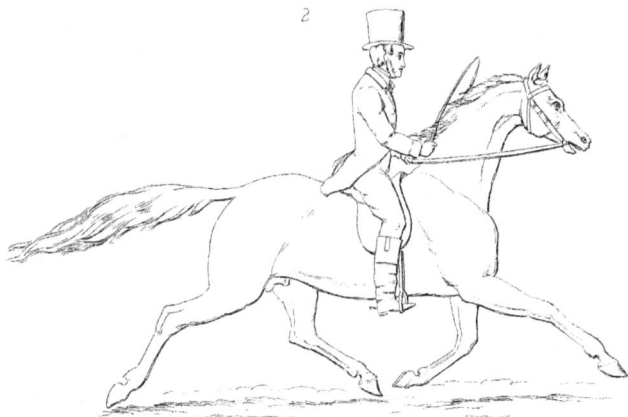

Road Riding

fore hand by drawing the lower finger on each side rather upwards and towards the body, avoiding all jerks or sudden motions.

During the trot he must sit close to the saddle, preserving his seat by the balance of his body, and not by the pressure of his knees; he must neither rise nor stand in the stirrups; his body must incline a little backwards; the whole figure must partake of and accompany the movements of the horse; and he must keep the hands up in their proper situation, steady and pliant, preserving a due correspondence, and just appuy. If the action be too rapid, it must be checked by strengthening the hand. If the action be too slow, it may be quickened by easing the fingers, and giving more animation.

To give more animation, and encourage the horse to put his foot out freely, the rider must support his fore hand up, and his haunches under, by a touch of the fingers, the excitement of the tongue, the switch of the whip, or the application of the legs, varied so as not to lose their effect. If the action be not sufficiently united, that also must be corrected.

To unite the horse, the reins must be collected, and the head raised. By bringing his haunches under him, he may be pressed up to the bridle by the aid of the legs; care being taken that this is not done hastily or violently. He must not, however, be confined in the hand, in expectation of raising him, and fixing his head in a proper place, as by this means his bars and mouth would soon grow callous.

The most certain sign of a horse's trotting well is, that when, in his trot, the rider presses him a little, he offers to gallop. If the horse gallop when he ought not, the waist should be pushed forwards toward the pommel of the

16*

saddle, and a bend or hollow at the same time be made in the loins.

Turns, Stops, &c. in the Trot.

As to turns, seeing that the operations directed to be performed at the walk are to be practised in the trot, nothing further need be said of them. As stops are required to coincide with cadences, it must be observed that the first part of the cadence in the trot is performed by the two feet that lead; and that the conclusion of the cadence is performed by the two feet that follow, and this should complete the stop. The rider should occasionally alter the measure of the action, by strengthening the hand, and at the same time keeping up a sufficient degree of animation to prevent the horse from stopping. He may then give him liberty, and proceed with the same spirit as before. He may make a stop; and may even rein him back two or three steps; in both cases keeping him so united and animated that the instant the hand gives him liberty, he advances as rapidly as before. (Plate XXXIX. fig. 1.)

ROAD RIDING.

Road riding is here introduced, because the trot is its most appropriate pace.

The difference between manège and road riding consists chiefly in a shorter seat and a shorter stirrup being used in the latter. A certain freedom and ease are also admissible. These, however, must not exceed propriety, lead to neglect of the horse, or risk security. The hand should keep its situation and property, though the body be turned to any extreme for the purpose of viewing or conversing; and the body must not, by any freedom it takes, throw itself out of balance, or take liberties, when it cannot be done with safety.

When the trot is extended to an unpleasant roughness, the jolting may be eased by rising upward and slightly forward in the stirrups. The faster the horse trots, the easier it is to rise; for it is the action of the horse, and not any effort of the rider, that must raise him. The foot he leads with determines that which the rider must rise to; and, if the horse change his foot, he must change with him. He must accordingly rise and fall with the leading foot, rising when the leading foot is in the air, and falling when it comes to the ground. The rise and fall of the body are to be smooth, and as regular as the beats of the feet.

Though this is called rising in the stirrups, no great stress or dependence is to be put on them. Such improper use of the stirrups causes many persons to be thrown, by the horse shying or suddenly turning round. The rising of the body must not be accompanied by any motion of the arms, or lifting of the shoulders. The hand is to be held steady as well as low, to prevent galloping (which the forwardness of the haunches would render inevitable if the hand were either eased or lifted,) and the reins should be of that precise length which preserves as much correspondence as possible between the hand and mouth. The steadiness of the hand is also necessary for the support of the horse.

The slight inclination of the body permitted in road riding must not occasion any roundness in the back, which is invariably to be hollow, not only for appearance sake but for safety. The action of the body likewise must not cause the legs to move or press the horse, which might cause him to gallop. In trotting, the rider must pay the greatest attention to correct every propensity to lift, hitch, overrate, or gallop; and, whenever he feels these propensities, he must check them with the greatest nicety, in order not to retard the horse's speed. (Plate XXXIX. fig. 2, illustrates the Seat, &c., in Road Riding.*)

THE GALLOP.

As to the character of the gallop, when we press a horse in the trot beyond his capacity, or animate him with the legs while we raise or retain him with the hand, we compel him to lift his two fore-feet after each other, which commences the gallop. The near fore-foot is first raised from the ground; then the off fore-foot, which, however, passes the other, and they come to the ground in the same order, the near fore-foot making one beat, and the off fore-foot another, that being the most advanced or leading foot. The hind feet follow in the same manner; the near hind-foot marking a third beat, and the off hind-foot passing forward, and marking a fourth beat. Thus, when this pace is united and true, the feet mark a regular, sharp, and quick time of one, two, three, four. The perfection of the

---

* In road riding, the rule of taking the right hand of all you pass is well known; but there are some exceptions, which are thus noticed by Mr. Bunbury, in his ironical style :—

"In riding the road, should a man on horseback be in your way leading another horse, always dash by the led one; you might otherwise set the man's horse capering, and perhaps throw him off; and you can get but a kick or two by observing my instructions.—In passing a wagon, or any tremendous equipage, should it run very near a bank, and there be but a ditch, and an open country on the other side, if you are on business, and in a hurry, dash up the bank without hesitation; for, should you take the other side, and the horse shy at the carriage, you may be carried many hundred yards out of your road : whereas, by a little effort of courage, you need only graze the wheel, fly up the bank, and by slipping or tumbling down into the road again, go little or nothing out of your way."

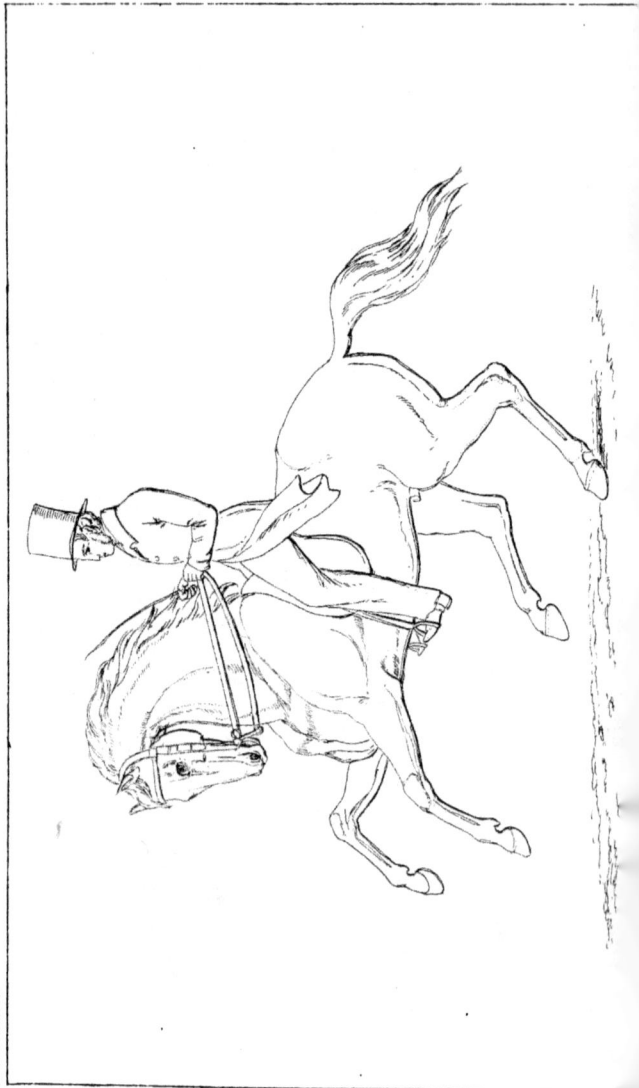

Plate XL

gallop consists in the suppleness of the limbs, the union of
the horse, the justness of the action, and the regularity of
the time.

The gallop is of three kinds—that of the racer, that of
the hunter, and that of the pleasure horse, commonly called
the canter. The last of these is by far the most difficult,
as it requires skill to fore-shorten and throw the horse on
his haunches. In the gallop, as in the trot, there is a leading foot. On a straight line, it is immaterial with which
fore-leg the horse leads, provided the hind-leg of the same
side follows it. But to lead always with the same leg is
injurious. In galloping to the right, the horse must lead
with the inward or off fore-leg, followed by the off hind-leg.
This action is termed true or united.—(Plate XL.* shows
this in the canter.) In galloping to the left, he must lead
with the inward or near fore-leg, followed by the near hind-
leg. This also is termed true or united.†

The Canter in Particular.

To put the horse to the canter from rest at any spot, or
from any pace, he must be pressed with the legs, or animated with the tongue, and at the same time, by a motion
of the fingers, and a little raising of the hand, be invited
to raise the fore-legs. If he do not obey this, the animation
must be increased, and the hand kept more firm, to pre-

* In galloping to the right, if the horse lead with the off fore-leg and
near hind-leg, or if he lead with the near fore-leg and off hind-leg, he
is said to be disunited. If, in galloping to the right, he lead with both
near legs, he is said to be false.

† In galloping to the left, if the horse lead with the near fore-leg
and off hind-leg, or if he lead with the off fore-leg and near hind-leg,
he is said to be disunited. If, in galloping to the left, he lead with
both off legs, he is said to be false.

vent his trotting; and this will constrain him to raise his
fore legs together. It is also necessary to direct the foot
he is to lead with. That of course is the inner, which he
will readily take by putting the croupe in, by means of the
opposite thigh, thereby enabling him to advance the inner
side.

As the position of the horse renders necessary a corresponding position of the horseman, it will readily be seen
that whichever side the horse leads with, the rider's thigh
on that side must be rather more turned in towards the
saddle, and the hip on that side brought more forward, and
consequently that the other thigh must be a little turned
outward, and the hip brought backward; and all this more
or less in proportion to the position of the horse. This turn
of the hip effects a turn of the body. The hands are carried with it, and at the same time kept up, rather above
than below the elbow, and quite steady, that the cadence
of every step, and the support given by the hand, may be
felt. The rider's head is of course to be directed to the
horse's nose, his eye glancing on the ground the horse's
fore-feet go over.

If the horse strike off with the wrong leg, false or disunited, the rider, at the first corner, must endeavor, by an
additional feeling of the inward rein, and application of the
outward leg, to make him change, and lead with the proper one. When he leads with the proper leg, the hand
must resume its usual position, the rider bending him a
little inwards by shortening the inward rein; the fingers
slackened, if necessary, to let him advance; but the hand
kept up, and every cadence felt of the fore-feet coming to
the ground.

There is far more skill displayed in keeping up an animated action in the canter, at the rate of three miles an

hour, than in the gallop, at that of twelve or fifteen. If the animation fail, or the action be not supported by the hand, the horse will break into a trot, particularly as the gallop is shortened or united. If the action is felt to be declining, it must be corrected instantly, by an animating touch of the fingers, the leg, or the tongue. The hand first discovers this declension, and is the first to correct it.

When the rider can put his horse off to either hand with the proper leg, and support the action, he must particularly attend to its truth and union, and try to raise it to the highest animation, riding sometimes rapidly, sometimes slowly, yet always united.

When the gallop is disunited and extended to speed, even though the horse is supple and just on his legs, it loses its harmony and regularity of time. The fore-legs then measure less space from each other, and so do the hind-legs, which makes the beats quicker in each, and leaves a space between the beats of the fore-legs and the beats of the hind. In these gallops, it would be highly imprudent to circle or turn, but on a very large scale.

Turns, Changes, Stops, &c. in the Gallop.

In turning the horse to the right and left, at a canter, his fore-hand must be raised with the leading rein, and the haunches pressed forward and under him : at the same time, the outward rein must assist to steady him, and a pressure of the calf of the outward leg keep the haunches from falling too much out. If he is turned suddenly with the inward rein only, without lifting the fore-hand, or applying the outward leg, he must turn on his shoulders, lose power to halt on his haunches, and being twisted round unprepared, will change to the outer leg.

In changing, the operation must be performed smoothly

and evenly at the same instant; so that, at the finish of the cadence, the body, hands, thighs, and legs of the rider are reversed, for the horse to commence his next cadence with the contrary leg.

In stopping in the gallop, the rider must seize the time when the horse's fore-feet are coming to the ground, which is the beginning of the cadence: and he must take care that the hind feet, coming up to their exact distance, and finishing the cadence, complete the stop: leaving the horse so balanced that he can readily set off again with the same rapidity as before. Besides seizing the exact time, a due degree of power must thus be exerted, conformably to the readiness, obedience, union, or rapidity of the action; for, should the power be deficient, the stop would not be properly effected; and if it be excessive, the horse will be over-balanced on his haunches, and compelled consequently to move his feet after the cadence is finished. Till horses are ready and obedient to the stop, it should not be attempted in violent and rapid gallops; nor even then if they are weak, or the rider heavy. In these cases, the double arret is used.

The double arret is the stop completed in two cadences of the gallop, which is far less distressing both to man and horse. The body being gently thrown back, will not make the action instantaneously cease; but the obedience of the horse makes the effort which checks half his career in the first cadence; and, the body still being kept back, he completes it in the second. However, till practised and made obedient to the stop, he will not easily perform the double arret; for, in the first instance, he must be taught to stop by compulsion; and it is only when practice has brought him to obedience, that he readily stops at the easy throwing back of the body.

Plate XLI

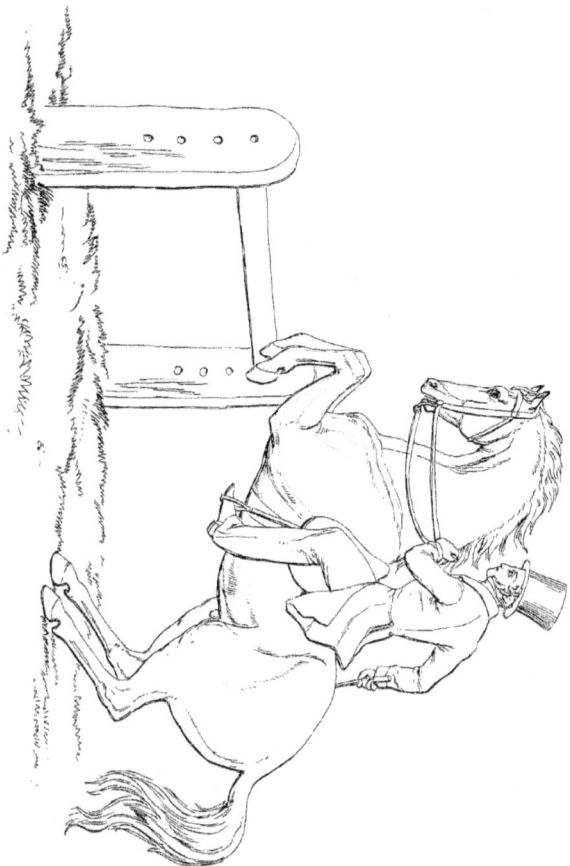

The Rise in Learning

The half stop is a pause in the gallop, or the action suspended for half a second, and then resumed again. Here the body is thrown back less determinately, lest we should so overbalance the horse that he cannot readily set off again after the finish of the cadence, which no sooner occurs than the body is brought forward, to permit the action to go on. Thus the half stop is only a pause in the gallop, and it is mostly used to effect a change from the right leg to the left, or the opposite. The cadence of the stop should be no shorter than the readiness and obedience of the horse will admit; the half stop not quite so short; and the two arrets still more moderate.

LEAPING.

The moveable bar for leaping should be ten feet in length, which will admit of two horses leaping abreast; at first from one to two feet high; and never very high.

As to the seat, it should be again observed that stirrups are no security in any situation on horseback; and those who cannot forbear pressing a weight on them, had better have none when learning to leap. An accurate balance must prevent all disturbance of the seat; for the slightest, whether the rider is thrown up from the saddle, or his body falls forward, or he gets out of balance, is as disgraceful as falling to the ground. He should sit so close as to carry a shilling under each thigh just above the knee, one in each stirrup under the toe, and one under his breech.

When any action of the horse tends to lift the rider from the saddle, stirrups cannot keep him down. Bearing on the stirrup, indeed, must lift the rider from the saddle, and would even loosen any hold he might take with the thighs or legs. Nothing but the weight of the body can press to the saddle. When the action is violent, however, the pres-

17

sure of the thighs may be employed to hold it down; and, when the hold of the thighs is not sufficient, the legs may take a deeper, and stronger hold. Leaps are taken standing or flying; the first being most difficult to sit, though always practised first, because the slow and steady leaping of a properly managed horse gives the rider time and recollection, and the riding-master an opportunity to direct, and to prevent accidents.

Standing Leap.

In the standing leap, the horse first shortens, and then extends himself. Readiness in the hand of the rider is therefore requisite to give the appropriate aids. These, if well timed, assist the horse: if otherwise, they check or embarrass him, and endanger both the animal and his rider. (Plates XLI. XLII. illustrate the Leap.)

The rider must therefore, by a ready and fearless yielding of the bridle, leave the horse at liberty to extend himself, preserving his own equilibrium only by leaning forward, as the horse rises, and backward as he alights. When he is brought to the bar, the body is to be upright. The legs are to be applied to his sides with such firmness as to keep the rider down to the saddle, and in such a manner—viz., perpendicularly from the knee—that the action of the body shall not loosen or disturb them. The toes must be pulled up, to make the muscles firm, and to prevent the spur from approaching too near the horse; and, if necessary, they may be turned out a little to strengthen the hold. The hand must be kept in the centre, and quite low; and the reins not too short, but just by the pressure of the fingers to feel the horse's mouth. When at the bar, the pressure of the legs and fingers will invite the horse to rise; and, as he rises, the body comes forward and preserves

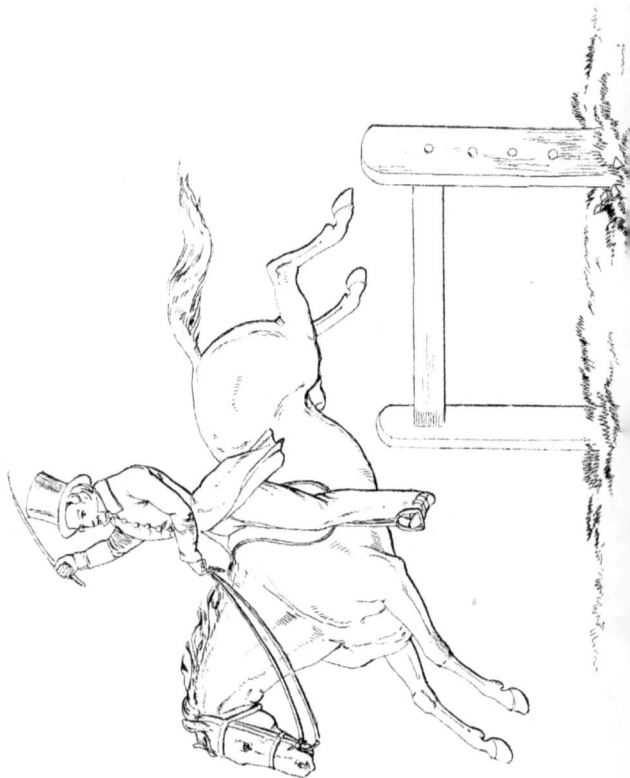

Plate XLII

its perpendicular. The back must then be kept in, and the head firm.

As the horse springs from his hind legs, and proceeds in the leap, the rider must slip his buttock under him, and let his body go freely back, keeping his hands down, legs close, and body back, till the horse's hind legs have come to the ground. The propriety of applying the legs to hold firm in the saddle is obvious. The hand being kept low is essential; and the bad consequences of raising it are numerous, as confining the horse, preventing the body going back, throwing the rider forward, &c.

The body coming forward to preserve its perpendicular as the horse rises before, prevents the weight of the rider from hanging on his mouth, and checking his leap, if not pulling him over backwards. The back being hollow when the spring forward is made, the body will of itself fall backward, if the hand be not raised to prevent it; and the head being firm may prevent a wrench of the neck, or a bite of the tongue. Slipping the breech under gives the body more liberty to lean back, and prevents the shock of the horse's feet meeting the ground, from throwing it forward.

While the seat is thus maintained, the hand must not be neglected. In riding up to a leap, the rider should yield the bridle to the horse, guiding him straight to the bar at an animated pace; halt him with a light hand, and upon his haunches; when he rises, only feel the reins to prevent their becoming slack; when he springs forward, yield the hand without reserve; and, when his hind feet come to the ground, again firmly collect him, resume his usual position, and move on at the former pace. If the horse be too much collected previous to his leap, he will bound, or buck over, as it is called. If not sufficiently collected or animated, he will probably not clear the leap. The degree in which a horse should be collected and animated depends on the temperament of the animal, and must be left to the judgment of the rider.

Flying Leap.

The flying leap is distinguished from the standing leap by its being made from any pace without a previous halt; and although the action is quicker, it is much easier. The pace, however, at which the rider goes at a flying leap, should always be moderate, in order that the horse may not rise too soon or too late.

A horse who rises too far from the bar seldom clears his leap, and risks straining by the effort to cover it; one who rises too near is likely to strike his knees against it, and throw his rider, or hurt himself. If a horse be indolent, and require animation, it is better to rouse his apathy by the spur just before his head is turned towards the leap, than while he is running at it. If he leap willingly, let him take his own pace to it, and he will spring from his proper distance, and give himself due velocity. Twelve yards from the leap, the rider may turn his horse to it in a trot; he will strike into a gallop; and, by a stroke or two before he springs, increase his velocity, if he perceive that the height he has to cover requires that exertion.

The seat in the flying leap is exactly the same as in the standing one; but, as the horse keeps a more horizontal position, it is easier. The rider, however, must not bring his body forward, at the raising of the fore legs, because the spring from the hind legs immediately follows, and the body not only might not get back in time, but, if the horse did not come fair, or refused to take his leap, and checked himself, the body, if forward, might cause the rider to tumble over his head. He should, therefore, keep his body upright; take hold with his legs; keep his hand down; and, as the horse springs forward, his body is sure to take the corresponding action of leaning back, particularly if he, at the instant, slip his breech under him, and bring his waist forward with an exertion proportioned to the spring the horse makes. He must also take care not to bring his body upright, nor slacken the hold with his legs, till after the hind feet have come to the ground.

In this leap the horse requires but little support or assistance from the hand till he is coming to the ground, when the hand aids in bringing the body upright, and in supporting the horse. The assisting and lifting a horse over leaps may be done only by experienced riders, and even by them only when he leaps freely and determinedly. Whips should not be used when the rider first practises leaping.

CRITICAL SITUATIONS.

When a horse is addicted to stumbling, rearing, kicking and bolting, plunging, shying and restiveness, the seat is maintained as in leaps; and the arms are held firm to the body, the hands kept up, and the reins separate, rather short than otherwise. By these means, the horse's head being raised, he can with less ease either rear or kick, because, for such purposes, he must have his head at liberty. It is fortunate that horses which rear high seldom kick, and *vice versâ*.

On these occasions the first operation of the rider is to separate the reins, &c. The body must be kept upright, but flexible, to repel every effort the horse may make; the balance must be preserved by the muscles of the thighs; the legs are to be kept near the horse, but not to grasp till absolutely necessary. When he lifts his fore legs, the breech must be thrust out behind, by which the rider is prepared if he rears. As the fore feet come to the ground, the breech must be slipped under, which prepares for his kicking or springing forward; the legs being then in a situation to grasp, and the hands to keep a firm hold. In all displays of vice, the rider should first see that the saddle or girths do not pinch the horse, that the bit does not hurt his lips by being too high in his mouth, &c.

Stumbling.

By the rider pressing his legs to the horse's flanks, and keeping up his head, he may be made to go light on his fore legs; and the same should be done if he actually stumble, so as to afford him instant assistance. Hence it is evident that the bridle should be of such length in the hand, that, in case of stumbling, the rider may be thus able to raise the horse's head by the strength of his arms and the weight of his body thrown backward. If the rein be too long, it is evident that, in effecting this manœuvre, the rider is in danger of falling backward as the horse rises. By thus pressing the legs to the horse's sides, he may be made to keep his haunches under him in going down hill, or may be helped on the side of a bank.

Rearing.

The principle danger in rearing is the hazard of the horse's falling backwards. When, therefore, he rises straight up, the rider must throw his body forward, giving him all the bridle. The weight of the body will oblige him to come down; and the moment that his fore feet are *near* the ground, and *before* he touches it, both the spurs must be given him as firmly and as quickly as possible.

Another mode of subduing him is, whenever the rider is aware of the horse's disposition to rear, to have the reins separated; and the instant he perceives him going to rise, to slack one hand and bend him with the other, keeping the hand low. This compels him to move a hind leg, and being thrown off his balance, he necessarily comes down with his fore feet. He should then be twisted round two or three times, to convince him of the rider's superiority, which confuses, baffles, and deters him from rearing to any dangerous height. To break horses of this dangerous vice, it has been sometimes expedient to leap from them, and pull them backwards. This so frightens them that they are wary of giving the opportunity again. It is, however, an expedient to be attempted only at a particular crisis, and by persons perfectly collected, active, and agile.*

* On this subject an anonymous writer, in answer to a query, says, "I would advise you by no means to try the experiment in question, either as operator yourself, or on your own horse. At all events, pray make trial first of the following prescription, which will in most cases be found an excellent preventive, if not a total cure, of the propensity complained of, and which has the advantage over the method respecting which you inquire, of being much easier and safer in its application, and, I may perhaps add, surer in its effects, and less expensive on the whole.

" Get a strong thick curb-bit, with a good deep port reversed—that is, the curve of the mouth-piece must project towards the outside of the horse's mouth, and not inwardly towards his throat, as in the common port bit. The thickness and exact curve of the bit should be calculated according to the size, strength, and hardness of mouth of the animal for which it is intended. For a very hard-mouthed horse, the bit should be made with a very deep port, and as thin as possible, consistently with the strength requisite.

" In nine cases out of ten I have found that confirmed rearers are tender-mouthed, and the habit has been probably induced by their being bitted and handled too severely. A martingale will be found a useful addition to the bit I have described. Its full efficacy can only be sufficiently appreciated by its being used several times, till the horse has become in some degree accustomed to it."

Kicking.

Horses apt to kick, either when they go forward or stand still, must be kept much together, or held in closely. When this is attempted, the hands, though fixed, must not pull at the horse, if he does not attempt to force the hand, and get his head, but leave him at liberty to go forward. If, however, he attempt to get his head down, which would enable him to kick with such violence as to throw himself, he may have the head confined up. This disarms him, and he makes a bolt from all-fours.

When a horse kicks, the rider must throw the body backward. It is an effective punishment to twist him round a few times for this fault. If this is done towards his weak or unprepared side, (for every horse has a favorite side,) astonishment and confusion will deter him from farther contention. In case of bolting, the rider must not exert one continued pull, but make repeated pulls until the horse obeys. Horses accustomed to be allowed to bear on the bit would not understand the steady pull as a signal to desist; and some would so throw up their heads as to deprive the rider of all power without dropping his hand, when the horse would drop his head. In that case, a second pull would find his mouth, and thus speedily his progress might be stopped.

Plunging.

In plunging, a horse gets his head down, cringes his tail between his quarters, sets his back up, swells his body to burst his girths, and, in this position, kicks and plunges till his breath can be held no longer—that is, till he makes six or eight plunges. To sit these is to cure them; and to do this, the rider must take a firm hold with his legs, and be mindful that the horse, in getting his head down, does not pull him forward. There is no danger of his rearing; and therefore the rider has only to keep his body back, and hold firmly with his hands, to prevent him throwing himself down.

Shying.

When a horse, either by shying or restiveness, springs to one side, or turns short round, the rider's security depends on strict conformity to the rules already laid down, as to not bearing on the stirrups; keeping the legs near to the horse, to be ready on these sudden and unexpected occasions to lay hold; and yielding the body to go with him.

When a horse is about to fly to one side, he may be stopped by his rider's leg being pressed on the side he would fly to, and by keeping his head high and straight forward, so as to prevent his looking towards the object he starts at, unless indeed it be something you desire to accustom him to the sight of, and then, whether you keep his face to it throughout, or avert it at first, and turn it gently towards it at last, great steadiness is necessary. When he curvets irregularly, and twists himself to and fro, his head should be turned to one side, or both alternately, without permitting him to move out of the track; and the rider's leg should be pressed against the opposite side. In this case he cannot spring on one side, because the pressure of the leg prevents him, nor will he spring to the other, because his head is turned that way, and a horse never starts to the side to which he looks.

Moreover, he will not fly back from anything, but go forward, if both legs be pressed against his sides. Thus he may be made to pass a carriage or other object in a narrow road; and here perseverance is especially necessary when the object is just reached, or partly passed, for if in the habit of going back and turning round when frightened, he will certainly do so when, if, by the hands slackening and

legs failing to press, he discovers that you are irresolute;
and this he would probably do at the most dangerous moment, when there was scarcely room for him to turn, and
the wheels might take him in the rear. To touch his
curb rein at such a moment would add to the confusion and
danger.

Restiveness.

The horse generally commences his attack by stopping,
turning short round, mostly to the right hand, as taking
the rider to the greatest disadvantage. He expects the rider
will oppose the opposite hand, designedly attacks the weakest, and is so prepared against its efforts that it is vain to
attempt them. It must be the rider's rule never to contend with the horse on that point on which he is prepared
to resist.

Instead, therefore, of attempting to prevent the horse
with his left hand, the rider must attack him with his
right, turn him completely round, so that his head is again
presented the right way, and then apply the whip. If he
turns round again, the rider must still attack his unguarded
side, turn him two or three times, and let the heel and spur,
if necessary, assist the hand, before he can arm or defend
himself against it.

If he still refuse to go the right way, the rider must take
care that he go no other, and immediately change his
attack, turning him about and reining him backward,
which the horse is easily compelled to do when he sets himself against going forward. In these contests, the rider
must be collected, and have an eye to the surrounding
objects; for restive horses try their utmost to place their
riders in awkward situations, by sidling to other horses,
carriages, the foot-pavement, the houses, &c.

In this case, the rider, instead of pulling him from the

wall, must bend his head to it, by which his side next the wall is rendered concave, and his utmost endeavors to do injury are prevented. The instant, therefore, that the rider perceives his horse sidling to any object, he must turn his head to that object, and back him from it.

There are some horses who fix themselves like stocks, setting all endeavors to move them at defiance. There, happily, their defence can in no way endanger the rider. It must, however, be converted to punishment. Let them stand, make no attempt to move them, and in a short space—frequently less than a minute—they will move off themselves.

When these various defences, however, are not powerfully set up, the general rule is to push the horse forward; and, for this purpose, at first to make use of the switch, as it alarms him least, for the spurs surprise a horse, abate his courage, and are likely to make him restive. Indeed, the application of the whip or spurs, except to shift the croupe, or give efficacy to the hands, is of little use; and to repeat either, to make a restive horse go forward, is certainly wrong. When passion possesses the rider, it prevents that concord and unity taking place which ever should subsist between the rider and his horse. He should always be disposed to amity, and never suffer the most obstinate resistance of the horse to put him out of temper. If the contest does not demand his utmost exertion of strength, he should be able to hum a tune, or converse with the same composure and indifference as though his horse were all obedience. By these means, the instant a horse finds himself foiled, he desists, having no provocation to contend farther, and is abashed at his own weakness. It is the absence of passion which, added to cool observation, makes the English the best riders and drivers in the world.

TREATMENT OF THE HORSE.

Stables are generally too dark and too hot. They should be kept quite cool, though without any draughts.

"A way," says De Beranger, in Helps and Hints, "of making the most of your horses, is to rise early in the summer, in order to do half your day's work before the heat of the day; for lying by the whole of the rest of the day, not only affords a traveller time and opportunity for examining what is worthy of being seen, but enables him to start with horses quite fresh, and to finish the remaining stage after sunset: not only will your horses go through their task with less labor in the cool of the evening, but you will find them travel more freely towards a resting-place, which darkness leads them to expect."

A horse ought not to be ridden a stage while in physic, nor on the day of its coming off. If he be pushed at first setting out on a journey, or be compelled to make long stages, or be deprived of his customary baits, he gets jaded, and every additional mile adds to his uneasiness. Moreover, at setting out in the morning, a well-kept horse is necessarily full of food, and consequently, until his great gut be properly emptied, brisk action occasions uneasiness or pain, which causes restlessness.

"When I travel on horseback," says the same writer, "I make it a rule to walk every seventh mile, be the roads ever so level; it affords a wonderful relief both to man and horse, and, instead of producing a loss of time, helps you on. When you dismount for such ends, always slacken your girths, slightly lift up the saddle to let a little air under it, and teach your horse (what he soon will learn) to walk briskly by your side, and keep the step with you, taking care to hold either of the reins lightly in your hand,

and without shifting it over the horse's head. Your steed will soon give you demonstrations of his gratitude, for he will be full of affectionate playfulness as he jogs along at your side, only to be rivalled by his willingness to let you mount after you have tightened the girths again. I need hardly tell you not to put your arm or wrist through a rein whilst walking or running by the side of a horse, for it is replete with danger. A good run with one hand on the horse's withers is pleasant, and greatly removes the stiffness of the joints so frequently occasioned by much riding; but the reins should be held between the fingers only, and rather loosely."

Hence, it follows that, although expedition be indispensable, the horse ought not to be put on his best pace at first, but considerably within it. Even this pace should be for a short space only; the reins should be loosened; the mouth played with; and if he do not evacuate, the pace may be repeated once more,—unless, indeed, he sweat much with the first, which is a sign of weakness, or that his dung is hard, and he requires purging.

While on the journey, the rider should be less attentive to his horse's nice carriage of himself, than to his own encouragement of him, and keeping him in good humor. Though generally he should raise his horse's head, yet when he flags in consequence of a long day or hard work, he may indulge him with bearing a little more upon the bit than he would in taking a mere airing exercise, or afternoon's canter in the Park. Keeping company with some other horseman facilitates a stage, by the emulation it excites; so that a dull animal, which one can scarcely get seven miles an hour from, will do nine or ten without fatigue when in company.

In road-riding, a picker is indispensable both in winter

18

and summer. In winter, it is necessary to relieve the sole when snow accumulates there. When, however, the traveller knows that snow is on the ground, he may avoid the trouble of dismounting, by previously ordering his horse's soles to be payed over with tar, or with tallow having no salt in it. At all times, when the roads have received fresh dressings, a picker is indispensable, because a loose stone is very liable to lodge in the hollow of the foot, and is dangerously driven backwards between the frog and the shoe, at every step the horse takes.

Pace and length of stage must be adapted to the heat of the weather in summer, and to the depth of the roads in winter; both seasons having the effect of knocking up the horse. In either case, a cordial promptly administered recovers him for the prosecution of his journey. The cordial readiest provided, and which should be kept at hand by the provident traveller, is in the form of a ball, and composed of aniseeds, ginger, carraway, of each, powdered, half an ounce, and mixed up with treacle and meal to the proper consistence. But good ale or porter, from one pint to a quart, made warm, operates sooner, and, upon emergency, is nearly as readily obtained as the ball.

Walking a horse the last mile, especially of a long stage, is a practice highly beneficial. As, upon setting out, we should not go off at the quickest pace, so upon coming in, we should not dash into our quarters with the perspiration streaming from each pore, in the mild season, nor covered over with dirt, in consequence of the pace, in wet weather. Even in winter, the perspiration flies from a strong horse, if in condition, upon coming in more sheltered places, and the practices he is then subjected to are commonly of such a nature as to cause disease in one way or another, in embryo, if not immediately.

The rider is greatly to be blamed who stands quietly by, or hides himself in the parlor, while his horse is brought in hot, stripped of everything, and led about to cool, in the draught of a gateway, or has the dirt washed off by plunging him in a horse-trough or pond, or his legs brushed in cold water in the open yard, while pailfulls, at the same time, are thrown over them; the consequence of all which is cough or colic, bad eyes, swelled legs, or inflammation of some vital part, which deprives the animal of life.

The horse should have a large and comfortable stall, and without any door behind him, a draught from which, by blowing up his coat, might expose him to cold. On coming in, after being coaxed to stale, he should undergo (in winter time in doors) a wisping all over with straw, beginning at the head, and proceeding to the neck and fore-quarters. His eyes, nostrils, &c., should also be cleansed with a sponge, and his ears rubbed. He should, at the same time, have before him a lock of sweet hay, in his rack, or a prickle, or the hand; and the rider should see whether he eats or not, whether he enjoys the wisping, and whether he chiefly evince a desire to lie down or a craving for food.

The girths having been already loosened, but the saddle still remaining on his back, his head should be turned to the rack, and his hind-quarters, legs, and belly, sheath and fork, wisped, and his feet picked clean and washed. After this, the saddle should be removed by sliding it back over the croupe; and the dressing be extended to the withers, back, and so completely all over the carcass, until it is dry. The saddle should be hung out, with the inside toward the sun; and when the panels have been duly aired and dried, they should be slightly beaten and well brushed.

If the horse refuse the first proffer of hay, the rider may

conclude that he has been pushed too much, as to time or length. If he still refuse his food, though the dressing be finished, he may be assured that his stomach is disordered, and he must be cordialed. In winter, a warm mash of malt is most eligible; but, if not at hand, a bran mash, with an admixture of oatmeal, and a quart of good ale, may be given. In summer, a cordial ball will restore the tone of his stomach, without increasing the heat of his body so much as a mash would. If he is not aged, nor inured to cordialing, a small pail of stout water-gruel, almost cold, excels all other cordials, and supersedes the necessity of watering; he will take his supper an hour or so afterwards, with a relish.

The traveller ought to look to every particular himself. In the next place, let him see that his horse gets his allowance of corn, that it be good, and that it contain no indications of having been in a manger before; for, in that case, he must wait by him until all the food is devoured. Dry food is alone proper to travel upon, and oats are the best; much hay being apt to engender flatulencies. When, however, a very long stage is to be taken, or it is cold, dreary, wet, or windy, a handful of crushed beans sustains him admirably, staying by him, and imparting vigor for a long time. The horse should not be denied water often; though too much at one time should not be given, nor, without its being chilled, any immediately after being fed.

His feet and shoes should be looked to, to ascertain if aught require repair, in order that it may be furnished as soon as he has recovered from his fatigue. His limbs, moreover, should be examined all over, for cracks, pricked foot, &c., and the body, for saddle-galls, &c. Now, as ever, his dunging should be looked to. Even if in full condition, having been well and regularly fed, and as regularly worked, he will contract a tendency to constipation ; the least ill consequence of which is defective pace, or short step, arising from more labored action. As the inconvenience may be suffered to last, he sweats immoderately at the least extra exertion, his eyes lose their wonted brightness, his mouth becomes hot, and his manner is languid. All these evils may be prevented by timely physicking, whenever the dung is seen to fall upon the ground without the pellets breaking. Even a little green food, or a day's mashing with bran, thin oatmeal gruel, and the like, will soften the dung considerably. It must be remembered that these things are to be undertaken on blank days, when the traveller is certain the horse will not be ridden a stage. The following allowance per week is generally enough to keep a horse in good condition :—

	Oats.	Beans.	Hay.
For a horse of from 14½ to 16 hands.	1¾ bushel.	2 quarterns.	1¼ truss.
For a horse under 14½ hands.	1½ bushel.	1½ quartern.	1 truss.

DRIVING.

Among the ancients, for more than one thousand years, the greatest honor that could be bestowed upon a man was a sprig of the wild olive tree entwined round his brow, for having gained a victory in the chariot-race at the Olympic games of Greece. This sprig of olive, moreover, was accompanied by other marks of distinction : the wearer of it was not only honored with statues and inscriptions. during his life-time, but the immortal Pindar, or some other great poet, was called upon to hand his name down to posterity in an ode. The Olympic games were revived, as a religious ceremony, by Iphitus, an Elean, about nine hundred years before Christ. They were celebrated near Olympia, in the territory of Elis. Horse and chariot races were considered their noblest sports. No one was there prevented from driving his own chariot; and kings were often seen contending against kings.

The Greeks were the most enlightened of the ancients, and their taste in the arts has never been even rivaled. What they did, therefore, on this occasion, could not be considered as in bad taste; and, when we remember that the celebration of these pastimes outlived the laws, customs, and liberty of their country, we need not say more in their vindication. The honors of victory were not even confined to the brave and skillful man who won the race; even the horses were crowned amidst the applauses of the spectators; and in one race, where forty chariots were broken, the victorious one was preserved in the temple of Apollo. Such being the havoc among the competitors, it is not wonderful that Ovid should say, that the honor of contending for the Olympic prize was almost equal to the winning of it.

Sophocles modestly speaks of ten starting at the same time in the race; but Pindar, availing himself, perhaps, of poetic license, makes the number forty. Four horses driven abreast was the usual number. The length* of the course on which they ran did not exceed an English mile, and as they had to make twenty-two turnings round the two pillars—generally, we may suppose, at full speed—

---

* The Circus Maximus at Rome, in which the Romans exhibited their chariot-races, was an oval building of one thousand eight hundred feet in length, and four hundred in breadth.

it is not difficult to imagine what dreadful accidents must have happened.

Nothing, indeed, but the form of chariot used could have ensured safety to any one. From the representations on ancient coins, it appears to have been very low, and only on two wheels, somewhat resembling our curricle. It had of course no springs; and, as there was no seat for the charioteer, much of his skill consisted in preserving his balance, and keeping upon his legs.

According to Pausanias, the following was the method of starting :—The chariots entered the course according to order, previously settled by lot, and drew up in a line. They started at a signal given, and to him who passed the pillar at the top of the course twelve times, and that at the bottom ten times, in the neatest manner, without touching it, or overturning his chariot, was the reward given.— As, however, it was the aim of every one who started to make for this pillar, as to a centre, we can easily imagine the confusion there must have been in forty, twenty, or even ten chariots, all rushing to one given point, amidst the clanging of trumpets, &c.

The following translation of a description of a chariot-race, from the Electra of Sophocles, is worthy of a place :

"When on the sacred day, in order next
 Came on the contest of the rapid car,
 As o'er the Phocian plain the orient sun
 Shot his impurpled beams, the Pythic course
 Orestes enter'd, circled with a troop
 Of charioteers, his bold antagonists.
 One from Achaia came ; from Sparta one ;
 Two from the Lybian shores, well practiced each
 To rule the whirling car: with these the fifth,
 Orestes, vaunting his Thessalian mares :
 Ætolia sent a sixth, with youthful steeds

In native gold arrayed: the next in rank
From fair Magnesia sprang: of Thrace the eighth
His snow-white coursers from Thesprotia drove:
From heaven-built Athens the ninth hero came:
A huge Bœotian the tenth chariot filled.
These, when the judges of the games by lot
Had fix'd their order, and arranged their cars,
All, at the trumpet's signal, all at once
Burst from the barrier; all together cheer'd
Their fiery steeds, and shook the floating reins.
Soon with the din of rattling cars was filled
The sounding hippodrome, and clouds of dust
Ascending, tainted the fresh breath of morn.
Now mix'd and press'd together, on they drove,
Nor spared the smarting lash; impatient each
To clear his chariot, and outstrip the throng
Of dashing axles, and short-blowing steeds,
They panted on each other's necks, and threw
On each contiguous yoke the milky foam.

" But to the pillar as he nearer drew,
Orestes, reining-in the nearmost steed,
While in a larger scope, with loosen'd reins,
And lash'd up to their speed, the others flew,
Turn'd swift around the goal his grazing wheel.

" As yet erect, upon their whirling orbs
Rolled every chariot, till the hard-mouth'd steeds
That drew the Thracian's car, unmaster'd, broke
With violence away, and turning short,
(When o'er the hippodrome with winged speed
They had completed now the seventh career,)
Dash'd their wild foreheads 'gainst the Lybian car.
From this one luckless chance a train of ills
Succeeding, rudely on each other fell
Horses and charioteers, and soon was fill'd
With wrecks of shatter'd cars the Phocian plain.

" This seen, the Athenian, with consummate art,
His course obliquely veer'd, and, steering wide
With steady rein, the wild commotion pass'd
Of tumbling chariots and tumultuous steeds.
Next, and though last, yet full of confidence

And hopes of victory, Orestes came;
But when he saw of his antagonists
Him only now remaining, to his mares
Anxious he raised his stimulating voice.
And now with equal fronts abreast they drove,
Now with alternate momentary pride
Beyond each other push'd their stretching steeds.
 "Erect Orestes, and erect his car,
Through all the number'd courses now had stood:
But luckless in the last, as round the goal
The wheeling courser turn'd, the hither rein
Imprudent he relax'd, and on the stone
The shatter'd axle dashing, from the wheels
Fell headlong; hamper'd in the tangling reins
The frighted mares flew diverse o'er the course.
 "The throng'd assembly, when they saw the chief
Hurl'd from his chariot, with compassion moved,
His youth deplored; deplored him, glorious late
For mighty deeds, now doom'd to mighty woes;
 Now dragg'd along the dust, his feet in air:
Till, hasting to his aid, and scarce at length
The frantic mares restraining, from the reins
The charioteers released him, and convey'd,
With wounds and gore disfigured, to his friends.
The just Amphictyons on the Athenian steeds
The Delphic laurel solemnly conferr'd."

In a political view, these games were productive of local
advantages; for, being sacred to Jupiter, they protected
the inhabitants of Elis against all the calamities of war.
In an economical point of view, they were of general use;
for, as Greece was generally short of horses, nothing was
so likely to encourage the breeding of them as the emulation thus raised among the different states. The circulation of money also was not a trifling consideration; for the
olive crown was obtained at great expense. By these games
being celebrated at the beginning of every fifth year, the
Greeks settled their chronology and dates; and as they

lasted a thousand years, a great part of the traditional history of Greece rests upon their base. That the honor of the prize was above all price, the following anecdote shows : —A Spartan having gained the victory at the Olympic games with much difficulty, was asked what he should profit by it ? " I shall have the honor," said he, " of being posted before my king in battle." As a further proof of the value and the moral effect of these contentions for honor, it is stated that, when a conqueror returned to his native city, he made his entry through a breach in the wall —by which was implied that cities inhabited by such men · had no need of walls.

A senator of Rome, indeed, says Gibbon, " or even a citizen, conscious of his dignity, would have blushed to expose his person or his horses in a Roman circus. There, the reins were abandoned to servile hands; and, if the profits of a favorite charioteer sometimes exceeded those of an advocate, they were considered as the effect of popular extravagance, and the high wages of a disgraceful profession." The Romans, with more pride, were far less intellectual than the Greeks ; but it must still be borne in mind, that, inconsistently enough, the interest taken in the charioteers of Rome shook the very foundation of the government.

In modern times, notwithstanding the sneers directed against gentlemen-coachmen and driving-clubs, it is to them chiefly that this country is indebted for the present excellent state of the roads, and for safe and expeditious travelling. The taste for driving produced, between men of property and those connected with the road, an intercourse which has been productive of the best results. Roadmakers, and those who have the care of roads, if they have not acted under the immediate direction of these amateur drivers, have been greatly benefited by their advice—

doubly valuable, as proceeding from knowledge of what a road ought to be. The intercourse also that has lately been carried on between proprietors of inns and of coaches, and gentlemen fond of driving, has greatly tended to direct the attention of the former to the accommodation and comfort of travellers. The improvement in carriages—stage-coaches more especially—would never have arrived at its present height, but for the attention and suggestions of such persons.

Moreover, the notice taken by gentlemen of coachmen, who are at once skillful and who conduct themselves well, has worked the reformation which has been of late years witnessed in that useful part of society.

Gentleman-driving, however, has received a check, very few four-in-hands being visible. The B. D. C., or Benson Driving Club, which now holds its rendezvous at the Black Dog, Bedfont, is the only survivor of those numerous driving associations whose processions used, some twenty years ago, to be among the most imposing, as well as peculiar spectacles in and about the metropolis.*

THE ROADS.

The excellence of our present mail-coach work reflects the highest credit on the state of our roads. The hills on great roads are now cut triangularly, so that drivers ascend nearly all of them in a trot. Coachmen have found out that they are gainers here, as, in the trot, every horse does his share, whereas, very few teams are all at work together when walking.

As, however, dreadful accidents have occurred to coaches

* The reader will bear in mind that this is many years after date. The R. D. C., which is now in the "Crescent," promises an ascendant of no mean effulgence.—ED. Fifth Edition.

when descending hills, a very simple expedient has been
suggested, by which these accidents may be avoided.   It
is merely a strip of gravel, or broken stone, about one yard
wide, and four or five inches deep, left on the near side of
the hill, and never suffer to bind or diminish.   This would
afford that additional friction (technically called a bite) to
the two near-side wheels, so that the necessity of a drag-
chain (never to be trusted) would be done away with, and
even in case of a hame-strap or pole-chain giving way, one
wheel-horse would be able to hold back a coach, however
heavily laden.   No inconvenience to the road, it is observed, could arise from this precaution, as carriages ascending the hills would never be required to touch the
loose gravel, it not being on their side of the road.   This
has been objected to, because some of the loose stones
might find their way into the middle of the road.   But,
admitting this might be the case, a trifling attention on
the part of the surveyor would obviate the objection.   A
man might be employed every second or third day to rake
these stones back again.   At the same time, it is obvious
that the neat appearance of a road is not to be put in the
scale against the limbs and lives of the people —Some
more permanent contrivance than loose stones even might
be found.

CARRIAGES.

Of carriages, those with two wheels are the cheapest,
lightest, and most expeditious; but, however sure-footed
the horse, and however skillful the driver, they are comparatively dangerous vehicles.

As to gentlemen's carriages, in this country, it has justly
been observed, that the view at Hyde Park Corner, at any
fine afternoon, in the height of the London season, is

enough to confound any foreigner, from whatever part of the world he may come. He may there see what no other country can show him. Let him only sit on the rail, near the statue, and in the space of two hours he will see a thousand well-appointed equipages pass before him to the Mall, in all the pomp of aristocratic pride, in which the horses themselves appear to partake. The stream of equipages of all kinds, barouches, chariots, cabriolets, &c., and almost all got up "regardless of expense," flows on unbroken until it is half-past seven, and people at last begin to think of what they still call dinner. Seneca tells us that such a blaze of splendor was once to be seen on the Appian Way. It might be so—it is now to be seen nowhere but in London.

As to stage-coaches, their form seems to have arrived at perfection. It combines prodigious strength with almost incredible lightness; many of them not weighing more than about 18 cwt., and being kept so much nearer the ground than formerly, they are of course considerably safer. Nothing, indeed, can be more favorable to safety than the build of modern coaches. The boots being let down between the springs, keep the load, and consequently the centre of gravity, low; the wheels of many of them are secured by patent boxes: and in every part of them the best materials are used. The cost of coaches of this description is from £130 to £150; but they are generally hired from the maker at $2\frac{1}{2}d.$ to $3d.$ per mile.

It is said to be the intention of Government* to substitute light carriages with two horses for the present mail-coaches drawn by four. On this, a writer in the *Quarterly Review* observes, that when the mail-coach of the present

---

* The era of railroads has however now arrived, and there remains no need for such an experiment.—ED. Fifth Edition.

day starts from London for Edinburgh, a man may safely bet a hundred to one that she arrives to her time; but let a light two-horse vehicle set out on the same errand, and the betting would strangely alter. It is quite a mistaken notion that a carriage is less liable to accidents for being light. On the contrary, she is more liable to them than one that is laden in proportion to her sustaining powers. In the latter case, she runs steadily along, and is but little disturbed by any obstacle or jerk she may meet on the road: in the former, she is constantly on "the jump," as coachmen call it, and her iron parts are very liable to snap.

It may in this place be observed, that no stage-coach should be permitted to travel the road with wheels secured only by the common linchpin. It is in consequence of this that innumerable accidents have happened to coaches from wheels coming off; and in these improving and fast times, such chances should not be allowed to exist. It may not be uninteresting to the uninitiated to learn from the same clever and experienced writer how a coach is worked. Suppose a number of persons to enter into a contract to horse a coach eighty miles, each proprietor having twenty miles; in which case he is said to cover both sides of the ground, or to and fro. At the expiration of twenty-eight days a settlement takes place, and if the gross earnings of the coach be £10 per mile, there will be £800 to divide between the four proprietors, after the following charges have been deducted, viz., tolls, duty to government, mileage (or hire of the coach to the coach-makers,) two coachmen's wages, porters' wages, rent or charge of booking-offices at each end, and washing the coaches. These charges may amount to £150, which leaves £650 to keep eighty horses, and to pay the horse-keepers for a period of twenty-eight days, or nearly £160 to each proprietor for the

expenses of his twenty horses, being £2 per week for each
horse.   Thus it appears that a fast coach properly appointed cannot pay, unless its gross receipts amount to £10
per double mile; and that even then the proprietor's profits
depend on the luck he has with his stock.

COACH-HORSES.

A great change has lately taken place as to the English
coach-horse; and this is the foundation of many other accompanying changes.   Fifty years ago, the putting a
thorough-bred horse into harness would have been deemed
preposterous.   In the carriages of gentlemen, the long-
tailed black, or Cleveland bay—each one remove from the
cart-horse—was the prevailing sort; and six miles an hour
was the extent of the pace.   Now, however, this clumsy-
barreled, cloddy-shouldered, round-legged animal, something between a coach and a dray horse, as fat as an ox,
and, with all his prancing at first starting, not capable of
more than six miles an hour, and rendered useless by a
day's hard work, is no more seen ; and, instead of him, we
find a horse as tall, deep-chested, rising in the withers,
slanting in the shoulders, flat in the legs, with more
strength, and with treble the speed.

The animal formerly in use cost from 30*l*. to 50*l*.—Two
hundred guineas is now an every day price for a cabriolet
horse; and 150 guineas for a coach-horse, for a private
gentleman's work.   A pair of handsome coach-horses, fit
for London, and well broken and bitted, cannot be purchased
under 200 guineas; and even job-masters often give much
more for them to let out to their customers.   The origin
of this superior kind of coach-horse is still, however, the
Cleveland bay, confined principally to Yorkshire and Dur-
ham, with perhaps Lincolnshire on one side, and Northum-

berland on the other, but difficult to be met with pure in either county. Cleveland indeed, and the Vale of Pickering, in the East Riding of Yorkshire, are the best breeding counties in England for coach-horses, hunters, and hackneys.

When the Cleveland mare is crossed by a three-fourth or thorough-bred horse of sufficient substance and height, the produce is the coach-horse most in repute, with his arched crest and high action. From the same mare and the thorough-bred of sufficient height, but not of so much substance, we obtain the four-in-hand, and superior curricle horse. From less height and more substance, we derive the hunter, and better sort of hackney. From the half-bred, we have the machiner, the poster, and the common carriage-horse.

The best coach-horse is a tall, strong, over-sized hunter. The hackney has many of the qualities of the hunter on a small scale. There is some deception, however, even as to the best of these improved coach-horses. They prance nobly through the streets, and they are capable of more work than the old clumsy, sluggish breed, but still they have not the endurance that is desirable ; and a pair of poor post horses, at the end of the second day, would beat them hollow.

In this carriage-horse, the bending of the upper joints, and the consequent high lifting of the feet, are deemed an excellence, because they add to the grandeur of his appearance; but this is necessarily accompanied by much wear and tear of the legs and feet, the effect of which is very soon apparent. The most desirable points in the coach-horse are—substance well placed, a deep and well-proportioned body, bone under the knee, and sound, open, tough feet.

One part of the old system, however, remains—namely,

that although little horses, well bred, are the fashion, large horses are still employed in heavy work. It must indeed be so. Horses draw by their weight, and not by the force of their muscles, although these, by carrying forward the centre of gravity, assist the application of that weight. It is the weight of the animal which produces the draught, and the power of the muscles serves to direct it. The hind feet form the fulcrum of the lever by which this weight acts against a load, and the power exerted is in proportion to the length of the lever, if the weight remains the same. Large animals, therefore, draw more than small ones, though they may have less muscular power, and are unable to carry weight so well. Nothing can better show that horses draw by their weight than the frequent occurrence that a horse is unable to draw a cart out of a slough until a sack of corn is thrown on his back, when he has little difficulty in doing it. Thus it is, that what are technically called lobbing-goers take more weight with them than horses of better action.

As the application of the weight or force proceeds from the fulcrum formed by the hind feet, good hind legs and well-spread gaskins are essential points in a coach-horse.— We even sometimes see that a wagon-horse, when brought to pull, will not touch the ground at all with his fore-feet. Another reason why little horses are unfit for heavy work is, that they will seldom walk and draw at the same time; for if they walk, they catch at their collars, and do but little. They never take anything like an even share of draught.

By calculations as to the mean strength of animals, it appears that a horse drawing horizontally, and at the rate of two miles and a half an hour, can work for eight hours in succession against a resistance of 200 pounds. If that pace be quadrupled, he finds an eighth part of the time sufficient. Thus we can pretty nearly measure a horse's power in harness. Whether we are carrying supposed improvement too far, and sacrificing strength and endurance to speed, is a question not difficult to be resolved.

A horse at a pull is enabled, by the power and direction of his muscles, to throw a certain weight against the collar. If he walk four miles in the hour, part of the muscular energy is expended in the act of walking; and consequently, the power of drawing must be proportionally diminished. If he trot eight miles in the hour, more of that energy is expended in the trot, and less remains for the draught; but the draught continues the same, and, to enable him to accomplish his work, he must exert his energies in a degree so severe and cruel, that it must speedily wear him out. Hence, there is no truth so easily proved, or so painfully felt by the postmaster, as that it is the pace that kills. Moreover, many a horse used on our public roads is unable to employ all his natural power, or to throw his weight into the collar, in consequence of being tender-footed, or lame. Being bought, however, at little price, he is worked on the brutal principle that he may be "whipped sound!"—and so he is apparently. At first he sadly halts, but, urged by the torture of the lash, he acquires a peculiar mode of going. The faulty limb keeps pace with the others, but no stress or labor is thrown upon it; and he gradually contrives to make the sound limbs perform among them all the duties of the unsound one. Thus he is barbarously "whipped sound," and cruelty is for the time undeservedly rewarded. After all, however, what is done? Three legs are made to do that which was almost too much for four. Of course, they are most injuriously strained, and quickly worn out; the general power of the animal is rapidly exhausted; and, at no remote time, death releases him from his merciless persecutors.

Happily, art is doing what humanity refuses. Railroads are rendering draught comparatively easy. An instance has been described of the power of a horse when assisted by art, as exhibited near Croydon. The Surrey iron railway being completed, a wager was laid that a common horse could draw thirty-six tons for six miles along the road, drawing his weight from a dead pull, and turning it round the occasional windings of the road. A numerous party assembled near Merstham to see this. Twelve wagons loaded with stones, each wagon weighing about three tons, were chained together, and a horse taken promiscuously from a timber cart, was yoked to the train.— He started from a house near Merstham, and drew the chain of wagons with apparent ease almost to the turnpike at Croydon, a distance of six miles, in one hour and forty-one minutes, which is nearly at the rate of four miles an hour. In the course of the journey he stopped four times, to show that it was not by any advantage of descent that his power was facilitated; and, after each stoppage, he again drew off the chain of wagons with great ease. A person who had wagered on the power of the horse then desired that four more loaded wagons should be added to the cavalcade, and with these the same horse set off again with undiminished pace. Still further to show the effect of the railway in facilitating motion, the attending workmen, to the number of fifty, were directed to mount on the wagons, and the horse proceeded without the least distress. Indeed, there appeared to be scarcely any limit to the power of his draught. After this trial, the wagons were taken to the weighing-machine, and it appeared that the whole weight were as follows :—

	tons.	cwt.	qrs.
12 wagons first linked together . . .	38	4	2
4 ditto, afterwards attached . . .	13	2	0
Supposed weight of fifty laborers . . .	4	0	0
	55	6	2

It is fortunate for breeders of horses that a perfect form
is not necessary to a good coach-horse. Some of those,
indeed, which the London dealers sell at high prices for
gentlemen's work, are such brutes, when out of harness,
that no man would ride them for their worth. The strong
and lengthy shoulder, with well-bent hind legs, are not absolutely necessary; and a good head and tail, with a little
high action, are all that is essential.

The following are useful hints for purchasers of coach-
horses:

No gentleman should purchase a horse without a good
trial of his mouth and temper. To be perfect in the first
respect, he should be what is called on the road "a cheek
horse,"—that is, should require very little curb, should
always be at play with his bit, and yet not afraid of it, and
should have each side of his mouth alike. To a gentleman's
leader, a good mouth is most essential, and then, the higher
his courage, the safer he is to drive. With stage-coach
horses, mouth is not of so much consequence, because they
are always running home, and there is no turning and
twisting, as in gentlemen's work, which is often in a crowd.
A whistle, or a click with the tongue, should make a gentleman's leader spring to his collar in an instant: one that
requires the whip should be discharged.

With wheel horses, which are steady and hold well, a
coachman may almost set his leaders at defiance; but if
they are otherwise, danger is at hand. It is not a bad plan

to purchase wheelers out of coaches, after they have been about six months in regular work. For from sixty to eighty guineas, the best of any man's stock may be picked; and a sound, well-broke coach-horse is not dear at that price. The coach-horses of gentlemen should be high in flesh, as it enhances their appearance, and is no obstacle to pace. A sound five-year-old horse, with good legs and feet, and driven only in harness, will last, on an average, from six to ten years in gentlemen's work, and will afterwards be very useful for other purposes.

The average price of horses for fast stages is about 23*l.* Fancy teams, and those working out of London, may be rated considerably higher; but, taking a hundred miles of ground, well horsed, this is about the mark. The average period of each horse's service does not exceed four years in a fast coach—perhaps scarcely so much. In a slow one, it may extend to seven. In both cases, horses are supposed to be put to work at five or six years old. The price named as the average may appear a low one; but blemished horses find their way into coaches, as do those of bad temper, &c. As no labor, while it lasts, is harder than that of coach-horses in fast work, it is wrong to purchase those which are infirm, as many proprietors do. Generally speaking, such horses are out of their work half their time, and are certain to die in their owner's debt. As the roads now are, blind horses are less objectionable than infirm ones. A blind horse that goes up to his bit, is both pleasanter and safer to drive than one with good eyes that hangs away from his work. Blind horses, however, work best in the night.

A horse cannot be called a coach-horse unless he has good legs and feet. As a wheel-horse, he is never to be depended upon down hill, if he has not sound limbs. He

cannot resist weight, if he be weak in his joints. To bad
legs and feet are owing numerous accidents to coaches,
many of which the public hear nothing of. If horses, on
the contrary, have good legs and feet, they will last, even
in the fastest work, many years, provided they are shod
with care, and well looked after. Proprietors of coaches
have at length found out that it is their interest to be hu-
mane and liberal to their horses, because the hay and corn
market is not so expensive as the horse market. They
have, therefore, one horse in four always at rest; in other
words, each horse lies still on the fourth day. Generally
considered, perhaps, no animal toiling solely for the profit
of man, leads so comfortable a life as the English coach-
horse: he is sumptuously fed, kindly treated, and if he
does suffer a little in his work, he has mostly twenty-three
hours in the twenty-four of perfect ease; he is now almost
a stranger to the lash, nor do we ever see him with a broken
skin. No horse lives so high as a coach-horse. Hunters,
in the hunting season, do not eat the quantity of corn that
coach-horses do; for the former are feverish after their
work, which is not the case with the latter, as they become
accustomed to this almost daily excitement. In the lan-
guage of the road, the coach-horse's stomach is the measure
of his corn—he is fed *ad libitum*.* The effect of this is,
that he soon gathers flesh, even in this severe work,—for
there is none more severe while it lasts: and good flesh is
no obstacle to speed, but the contrary.

It is not found, however, that (barring contagious diseases) where their owners are good judges of condition,
coach-horses are much subject to disease. After a hot

---

* Some coachmasters give their horses all manger-meat; but this is
wrong, as it often produces indigestion and disease. A certain portion
of long hay is necessary.

summer, coach-horses are most liable to derangement; and
the month of October is the worst in the year for them, in
consequence of it being their moulting season. Coach-
horses, indeed, are certain to sweat three days out of four,
which keeps their blood pure, and renders almost unnecessary medicine, of which, in general, they have but a small
portion—perhaps less than they should have. It is a mistake, however, that fleshy horses cannot go fast in harness;
they are more powerful in draught than thin ones; and,
having only themselves to carry, flesh does not injure their
legs, as in riding. In a fast coach, then, a horse ought
not to work more than four days without rest, as he becomes leg-weary, and wears out the sooner; and he becomes
also too highly excited. A horse a mile, reckoning only
one side of the ground, is about the proportion. Thus we
may suppose that ten horses work the coach up and down
a ten-mile stage, which gives eight at work, and two at rest.
Every horse, then, rests the fourth day. In slow, heavy
work, however, coach-horses will do their ground every
day, barring accidents or illness.

In slow work, the average duration of coaching stock may
be from six to seven years, provided they are at first fresh,
and firm on their legs. In fast work their time may be
from three to four years, or scarcely perhaps so much.
Coach proprietors on a large scale should have a break for
their young horses, previous to going into regular work.
The practice of putting a young horse unaccustomed to
harness into a coach laden with passengers, is most reprehensible; and when injury is sustained by it, it should be
visited by the severest penalties the law can inflict.

HARNESS.

In the manufacture of harness we have arrived at a degree of perfection, to which the invention of the patent shining leather has mainly contributed. A handsome horse well harnessed is a noble sight; yet in no country, except England, is the art of putting a horse into harness at all understood. If, however, our road horses were put to their coaches in the loose awkward fashion of the continental people, we could not travel at the rate we do. It is the command given over the coach horse that enables us to do it.

In regard to mails, it should be observed that the proprietors who horse them are not sufficiently attentive to the state of the harness on the ground worked by night; whereas it should in reality be the best. If anything break by daylight, it is instantly observed; but it is not so in the night, as lamp-light is uncertain and treacherous. In speaking of particulars, it may be observed, that bearing-reins are a relief to the arm of the driver, but by no means to the horses. Indeed, they materially lessen the power of horses in drawing, become insufferable to them in a long journey, and fatigue them much sooner than they would otherwise be. Not only do these reins by no means serve to keep horses up, but they prevent their rising after having fallen.

When a wheel-horse has the habit of throwing up his head, which greatly annoys the mouth of the leader before him, a nose-martingale should be used. This, however, is rarely sufficient. Indeed, it is a bad custom to run the leader's reins through terrets over the heads of the wheelers; for then every movement which the wheelers make with their heads, acts powerfully on the mouths of the leaders, whether they be good or bad. If the former, it is sometimes attended with danger: thus, a wheeler throws up his head, suddenly and powerfully shortens the rein of the leader, who is checked, and as the wheeler goes on, he brings the bar with force against the hocks of the leader, which instantly flies forward, and mischief ensues.

This, perhaps, does not last long; but one evil only takes the place of another: leaders soon learn to be, from custom, equally heedless of this check and of their driver's hand: and their mouths become steeled by the constant tossing of the wheeler's heads. It is thus that we sometimes hear of leaders choosing their own road in spite of the best efforts of good coachmen; and so it will always be till terrets are totally abolished. This may easily be done by conducting the leader's rein through the rosette in which the wheeler's outside bearing-rein, of which we have just disapproved, at present passes, and thus supersede the terret.

Terrets, however, are supposed to look well, and to have the advantage of keeping the head steady. To obviate their disadvantages, therefore, in some measure, rollers are placed in the bottom of each terret, over which the rein passes. This, in some degree, obviates the evil, as the rein no longer holds in the terret, but slides easily, giving the wheeler's head more freedom. In all kinds of work, a tool-book is a necessary appendage to the coach. It should contain a strong screw-wrench, wheel and spring clips, a spring shackle or two, with bolts and nuts, and two chains —one for a trace, and the other shorter, with a ring at one end and a hook at the other, in case of a tug giving way. In his pocket the coachman should have a short strap with a buckle at each end, as in case of almost any part of the reins, or indeed most parts of the harness breaking, it comes into use in a moment.

The following are interesting extracts on this subject, from an article in a late number of the *Quarterly Review;* and the work quoted and referred to in the article is en-

20

titled Bubbles from the Brunnens of Nassau. "With regard to the management of horses in harness, perhaps the
most striking feature to English eyes is, that the Germans
intrust these sensible animals with the free use of their
eyes. 'As soon as, getting tired, or, as we are often apt
to term it, lazy, they see the postilion threaten them with
his whip, they know perfectly well the limits of his patience,
and that after eight, ten, or twelve threats, there will come
a blow. As they travel along, one eye is always shrewdly·
watching the driver; the moment he begins his slow operation of lighting his pipe, they immediately slacken their
pace, knowing as well as Archimedes could have proved,
that he cannot strike fire and them at the same time : every
movement in the carriage they remark; and to any accurate observer who meets a German vehicle, it must often
be perfectly evident that the poor horses know and feel,
even better than himself, that they are drawing a coachman, three bulky baronesses, their man and their maid,
and that to do this on a hot summer's day is no joke.'

"Now, what is our method? 'In order to break-in the
animal to draught, we put a collar round his neck, a crupper under his tail, a pad on his back, a strap round his
belly, with traces at his sides; and, lest he should see that,
though these things tickle and pinch, they have not power
to do more, the poor intelligent creature is blinded with
blinkers, and in this fearful state of ignorance, with a g oom
or two at his head, and another at his side, he is, without
his knowledge, fixed to the pole and splinter-bar of a carriage. If he kick, even at a fly, he suddenly receives a
heavy punishment which he does not comprehend; something has struck him, and has hurt him severely; but, as
fear magnifies all danger, so, for aught we know or care, he
may fancy that the splinter-bar which has cut him is some

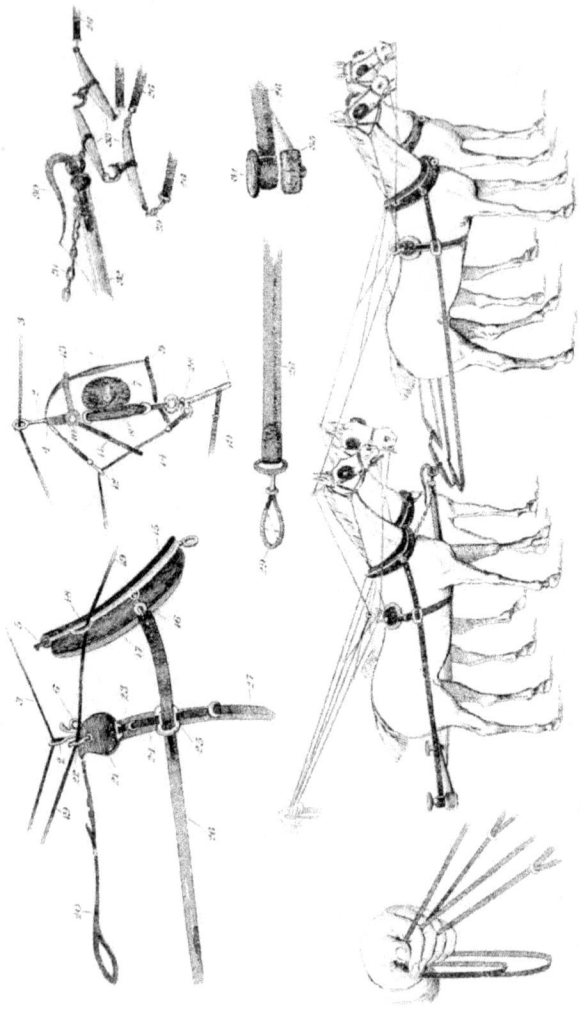

Plate XLIII

hostile animal, and expects, when the pole bumps against his legs, to be again assailed in that direction. Admitting that in time he gets accustomed to these phenomena—becoming, what we term, steady in harness, still, to the last hour of his existence, he does not clearly understand what it is that is hampering him, or what is that rattling noise which is always at his heels;—the sudden sting of the whip is a pain with which he gets but too well acquainted, yet the *unde derivatur* of the sensation he cannot explain—he neither knows when it is coming, nor what it comes from. If any trifling accident or even irregularity occurs—if any little harmless strap which ought to rest upon his back happens to fall to his side, the unfortunate animal, deprived of his eyesight, the natural lanterns of the mind, is instantly alarmed; and, though from constant heavy draft he may literally, without metaphor, be on his last legs, yet if his blinkers should happen to fall off, the sight of his own dozing master, of his own pretty mistress, and his own fine yellow chariot in motion, would scare him so dreadfully, that off he would probably start, and the more they all pursued him the faster would he fly."

DESCRIPTION OF PLATE XLII.

1. Face-strap,
2. Terret for the leader's rein.
3. Leader's rein.
4. Head-piece.
5. Hame-strap.
6. Bearing-rein hook.
7. Winker
8. Cheek-strap.
9. Nose-strap.
10. Rosette.
11. Throat-lash.
12. Bearing-rein roller.
13. Front piece, or fore-top.
14. Bearing-rein.
15. Hames.
16. Hame-tug.
17. Collar.
18. Hame-terret.
19. Wheeler's rein.
20. Crupper.
21. Pad.
22. Terret for wheeler's rein.
23. Belly-band.
24. Trace-bearer.

25. Trace-buckle.

26. Trace.

27. False belly-band.

28. Bit.

29. Swivel-hook.

30. Pole-hook.

31. Pole-chain.

32. Pole.

33. Shackle or swing-bars.

34. Tug.

35. Splinter-bar.

RELATIVE PLACES OF HORSES.

In placing horses in a team, we speak of near and off horses. The term of "near" is probably a borrowed one. In a wagon, the near horse is the one which is nearest the driver, who always walks with the horses to his right hand; and the other, running abreast of him, is called the off or far horse, because he is the farthest from the driver. This term, indeed, does not refer to coaching so well as to wagoning, as the coachman does not walk by the side of his horses; but many of the terms of coachmanship are drawn from the same source, and the expression "near" horse seems to be among the number.

The word "near" having been thus made use of in its original acceptation, has, in some counties, gradually superseded the world left, in contradistinction to right; as we hear occasionally of the "near side of the road," the "near wheel of a carriage," the "near leg of a horse;" in short, it is substituted for the word left. Or the term may have arisen intermediately from this: that on the first introduction of carriages into this country there was no driving on the box, but on the saddle, and that hence the term "near" was used to distinguish the saddle-horse, and the term "off," of course, the other horse. These terms were afterwards applied to the road, where, in meeting carriages, according to the adage, "If you go to the left, you are sure to go right;—if you go to the right you are wrong."

Wheel-horses have the hardest place, as they are at work up hill and down. Nevertheless, if favor be shown, it must be to the leaders, because a tired wheeler may be dragged home; but, in the road phrase, if a leader cuts it, you are planted. It is a rule always to put the freest leader on the near side, as he is better in hand than on the other. If a leader be weak, and cannot take his bar, the wheeler that follows him must be tied up, and this will place him by the side of his partner. Leaders should be fast trotters for fast coaches; for, if they gallop, the bars are never at rest, and consequently much of the draught is lost in the angles described. To a coach-horse in fast work, wind is almost as essential as to a hunter. Many high-blowers, however, keep their time very well, with a little attention on the part of the driver. If he see them distressed, he ought to keep them off their collar, and let them only carry their harness for a hundred yards or so, when they will recover, if their condition is good. They work best as night-horses; and, if driven in the heat of the sun, they ought to be out of the throat-lash. Indeed, a leader should never be throat-lashed in very hot weather, if he can be driven without it. Many horses pull, and are unpleasant in it, but go temperately out of it.

In coach-horses, temper is much to be regarded. Some contend that a horse should never know his place,—should go either wheeler or leader, and on either side. If, however, a horse working constantly in a coach prefer any place, he should have it, and he will generally pay for the indulgence. Some horses, indeed, care not where they are put working equally well or ill in all places. As to the mode of putting young horses in harness, the best way is to put one, for the first time, with only one other, which ought to be steady, good-collared, and quick. A great deal of room should be given his head, and he should be driven at the cheek of an easy bit, with his pole-piece rather slack. There is great want of judgment in throat-lashing a young horse—either wheeler or leader.

Many horses go perfectly quiet as leaders, that would never go as wheelers, because they will not bear being confined by the pole piece. All ought to have their sides frequently changed, particularly young ones. As to horses' mouths, some will not bear a curb chain at all, while the bars and chins of others are so hard, that it is difficult to make an impression upon them; the latter being most prevalent.

It is difficult, however, to handle a coach-horse, particularly a leader, whose mouth is very tender. A snaffle is not safe, as, in case of his dropping or bolting, it has not sufficient power to catch him up quickly, at such a distance from the driver's hand. For a gig horse, it may occasionally answer. The usual plan then is to "cheek him," as it is technically called, that is, to put his coupling-rein to the cheek instead of the bottom of the bit. Should this be severe for him, and he swing his head too much towards his partner, his draught reign should be put down to the bit, which will bring him straight. He should have liberty in his bearing-rein, and his curb-chain should not be tight. A check-rein to a nose-martingale is often of service in this case, as it keeps his head steady, and makes him face his work. Such horses in general, work more pleasantly out of the throat-lash.

Horses with very hard mouths require the bit with double port, the Chiffney bit, or the plan of putting the curb-chain over the tongue instead of under the chin, which in some prevents what is termed a dead mouth. Letting out the head of the bridle in the middle of a stage, has also considerable effect, as causing the bit and curb-chain to take hold in a fresh place. A check-rein likewise is sometimes put to the middle link of the curb-chain, to retain the bit in the middle of the mouth, and to keep it alive, as it is termed. In hard pullers, moreover, putting the bearing-rein to the *top*, and the coupling-rein to the lowest loop in the bit, creates a counter-action, not only making the bit more severe, but keeping the mouth in play. A hard puller is generally safest, and more in place before the bars than at wheel; for, with a good pair of wheel horses, leaders are soon checked, and he pulls less with a free than with a slack partner.

A coach-horse, if obedient to the hand, cannot well carry his head too high, while a horse that goes with his head down has a mean appearance in harness. The horse, however, that carries his head higher than his partner, should have his coupling-rein uppermost. A coach-horse should not be broken in a fast coach, as in fast work there is no time to try his temper, and to humour him. By being put at first into quick work, many horses get into a habit of cantering, and never trot well afterwards.

A kicking wheel-horse should be put on the near side, where he is less liable to be touched by anything that might annoy him; for, on the off side, throwing the reins on his back, or touching his tail when getting anything out of the boot, may set him off, and cause mischief. A kicking leader should have a ring on the reins, for many accidents arise by a leader's getting a rein under his tail, owing to the want of this. With first-rate coachmen, however, this precaution is the less essential, that they generally have their horses better in hand. With horses very fresh in condition it sometimes happens, especially in a turn, that a wheeler kicks over his trace, and an

accident is sometimes the consequence. A light hip-strap
prevents this, by taking the trace up with him when he
rises. In London, this is particularly useful; for, when
horses are turning short, or in a crowd, they frequently
have their traces slack, and therefore more easily kicked
over. The hip-strap looks slow, but it is safe.

COACHMEN.

Of late years, a superior class of men form our coachmen;
and for this we are mainly indebted, first, to the driving
clubs, and the notice taken of coachmen by men of fortune;
and, secondly, to the boxes being placed on springs. The
latter renders it a common practice for passengers to pay
an extra shilling for the box place, whereas formerly a man
would have given something to be anywhere else. We are
told that good coachmen are becoming, in proportion to
their number, more scarce every year, because owing to
the fine state of the roads, the condition of the cattle, and
the improved method of road work, coach-horses are so
above their work, that the assistance of the driver is seldom
required. " When in town," says a writer in the *Sporting
Magazine*, " I sometimes take a peep at the mails coming
up to the Gloucester Coffee-house; and such a set of spoons
are, I should hope, difficult to be found; they are all legs
and wings; not one of them has his horses in hand; and
they sit on their boxes—as if they were sitting on something else."

Certain it is that coach-work in perfection is not to be
seen a hundred miles from the metropolis—seldom so far.
The build of coaches, the manufacture of harness, and the
stamp and condition of horses are greatly inferior in the
northern counties; and as to the coachmen, few that at all
deserve the appellation. There are few things in which

knowledge of an art without execution is of less value than in driving four-in-hand; for, although a coachman may have knowledge, it is possible that, from natural awkwardness, he may be unable to put it into practical effect with a neat and appropriate movement of his arms and hands; and seldom is a certain propriety and neatness more required than in handling the reins and whip. To make a man a good driver, there is one requisite, and that is, what are called on the road, "hands,"—a nice faculty of touch. No man with a hard, heavy hand can ever make a good horseman or driver. Neither will a nervous man ever be safe on a coach-box, for presence of mind and strong nerve are there very often called into action.

The air and manner of a coachman have been cleverly described by some periodical writers. Let us, say they, suppose the horses put to their coach, all ready for a start —the reins thrown across the off wheel-horse's loins, with the ends hanging upon the middle terret of his pad, and the whip thrown across the backs of the wheelers. The coachman makes his appearance. If he be a coachman, a judge will immediately perceive it; for, as a certain philosopher observes, "every situation in life serves for formation of character," and none more so than a coachman's. I was going to say—only let a judge see him come out of his office, pulling on his glove; but this I will say—let one see him walk round his horses, alter a coupling-rein, take up his whip and reins, and mount his box, and he will at once pronounce him a neat, or an awkward one. The moment he has got his seat and made his start, you are struck with the perfect mastership of his art—the hand just over his left thigh, the arm without constraint, steady, and with a holding command, that keeps his horses like clockwork, yet, to a superficial observer, with reins quite

loose.   So firm and compact is he, that you seldom observe
any shifting, except perhaps to take a shorter purchase for
a run down hill, which he accomplishes with confidence
and skill, untinctured with imprudence.

In a coachman, temper is also one of the essentials to a
good workman.   We are told of a great artist, that, having
four "rum ones" to deal with, and being unable to make
them work to please him, he threw the reins on the footboard, and exclaimed, "Now, d—n your eyes, divide it
among you, for I will be troubled with you no longer."
The impertinences of passengers sometimes increase this
irritability.   In steam-vessels, they adopt the plan of
writing in large letters on the wheel which directs the
helm, "Do not talk to the helmsman."   It would be as
well in some coaches to have the same rule adopted—"Do
not babble to the coachman."

It is not possible to obtain a better idea of a good coachman, than from the following account of one who is said
to be the first coachman in England for bad horses.
"Having all his life had moderate horses—some strong
and heavy, some light and blood-like, old hunters, old
posters—most of the teams going and returning,—their
work at the utmost stretch, always overpowering,—having
also had always, besides difference in character, weak horses
to nurse,—this ordeal has worn him down to a pattern of
patience.   With these, and great weight upon severe
ground, he is steady, easy, very economical in thong and
cord, very light-handed and sometimes playful.   I observed
him closely, and discovered from his remarks, as well as
from what I saw, that his great secret of keeping his nags
in anything like condition, and preserving them when
apparently worn out, is by putting them properly together,
by constantly shifting their situations, and by the use of

check reins with remarkable judgment, by which means
he brings their powers as near to equality as possible,
besides preventing the evil of boring. Indeed, his horses
all go light and airy; and though at times his hold of
necessity becomes powerful, yet, generally speaking, he
takes his load without a severe strain upon his arms. I
own it is this particular knack which always wins me.
Both in driving and riding, give me the man who can
accomplish his object with a light hand."

The duty of a coachman is apt to injure the eyes—particularly in cold blowing weather. He must keep his eye
forward; and it is found that the sight cannot be fixed upon
anything beyond the head of the wheel-horses (not so far
as this, in short men,) without raising the eyelids, and consequently exposing the eyes to the weather. Six parts of
cold spring water, to one of brandy, is a good lotion when
the eyes suffer from this cause. Coachmen should also
preserve their feet and bodies from cold. In very cold
weather, the chin should be protected by a shawl, and the
knees by thick cloth knee-caps. In very severe weather,
the breast should be protected; for which purpose hare-
skins are now manufactured, and are getting into use on
the road.

A coachman ought not to drive more than seventy miles
a day; and, if this is done at two starts, so much the better.
The wearing of the frame, under daily excitement, must
tend to produce premature old age, and to shorten life; and
this excitement must be very considerable when a man
drives a fast coach eighty or a hundred miles a day without
a stop—particularly if his coach be strongly opposed.
Coachmen who wish to keep themselves light, take walking
exercise in their hours of rest from road-work.

As to amateur coachmen, it has been observed, that if a

diet were formed, before whom gentlemen-coachmen were to be examined previous to their being considered safe, it would not be amiss if they were put to the test of having the harness of four horses taken to pieces, strap from strap, and then requested to put it together again in the presence of the judges. There would be no hesitation in pronouncing him safe who succeeded in this, as his experience on the road must have been considerable. How these amateurs are trusted with the reins, coachmen are now obliged to be careful, owing to the speed of coaches, and the improved breed and condition of coach-horses. Hence, we see fewer amateurs at work than formerly. It would indeed be highly culpable in a coachman to trust the lives of passengers and his master's property to any one whom he did not know to be safe, or even without reflecting that a man may be a very safe coachman with horses he knows, and a very unsafe one on some roads with horses to which he is a stranger.

To gentlemen who wish to drive, and are really capable of doing so, the following is recommended as not a very bad way of doing business :—" When travelling with a coachman I do not know," says an amateur, "I always adopt the following plan—that is, if I wish to work. In the first place, I never got upon a coach-box yet with anything like half-pay about me ; such as a black handherchief around my neck, or in blue pantaloons ; neither do I think I ever shall. I always take care to have a good deal of drag about me :—a neat pair of boots, and knee-caps, if cold weather : a good drab surtout—if not a poodle ; a benjamin or two about the coach, and a little of the spot about the neck.— For the first mile, I always observe a strict silence, unless broken by coachee ; but at this time he generally runs mute. He is perhaps but just awake, or is considering about his way-bill—reckoning his passengers, thinking what he has to do on the road, and, if a workman, looking over his team to see if all is right. Leave him alone for a short time, and when his mind is at ease, he will look you over as you sit beside him. He will begin with your boots, proceeding upward to the crown of your hat, and if he like you, and you make a remark or two that please him, and show you to be a judge of the art, the first time he stops he will say—' Now, sir, have you got your driving gloves on ; would you like to take 'em ?'—I am here alluding to country work, and not to the roads near London."

Coachmen's expenses on the road being heavy, should be taken into consideration by passengers. They have their horse-keepers to pay every week, or they will not do their best for them; and the wear and tear of their clothes is a heavy tax on their pockets. They are satisfied, however, with one shilling under, and two shillings for anything over thirty miles; and they are well entitled to that sum—more especially when we recollect that they are liable to have empty coaches. No man, certainly, should give them less than a shilling, and if he often travel the same road, his money is not ill bestowed. In respectable coaches, no great difference is now made between the fees given by in and outside passengers, as it often happens that the latter is best able to pay.

Guards on mail coaches are necessary appendages to the establishment; and, that they may be equal to their duty, they go only moderate distances—as from sixty to eighty miles, when they are relieved by others. Those on the long stages, however, are imposed upon by their masters ; and, by being made to do more than they are equal to— many of them two nights up for one in bed, are half their time asleep. Some go from London to Exeter, Shrewsbury,

21

and other places equally distant, without stopping more than three quarters of an hour on the road, which, in bad weather, is hard enough. Indeed, it is wonderful how with their means they always contrive to live.

Guards are by no means useless appendages to stage coaches; for no coach, running a long distance and in the night, should be without one ; but such guards should be provided with fire-arms in good repair. Setting aside the idea of highway robbery, it is impossible that, in the night, a coachman can see to the luggage on his coach,—nor indeed, can the guard, if he be asleep, and asleep he must be a great part of his time, if worked in the way above stated. He should not go more than one hundred miles, and he should be paid by the proprietors. But if the public should not be left to pay an armed guard, it is monstrous that they should pay an unarmed one. As to mail-guards, government allows them only a mere pittance of a few shillings a week, leaving the public to pay them ; whereas the public have nothing to do with them, and it is the most impudent imposition that these servants of government should be paid by persons travelling. That they carry fire-arms is true ; but it is to protect the letter-bags —property which government is paid to protect—that they would use these arms, and not on account of passengers.— Strictly speaking, they have nothing to do with the passengers, nor their luggage ; their sole duty being to protect the mail. As, therefore, government is paid for carrying the mails, government, and not the public, should pay the persons who actually do protect them.

MOUNTING AND DISMOUNTING.

Before getting upon the box, a coachman should walk round his horses' heads, to see that his curb-chains and coupling reins are right, and above all, that the tongues of his billet-buckles are secure in their holes. Many accidents have arisen from the want of this precaution. No man is a safe coachman who does not see to these things. Of mounting and dismounting, there is nothing particular to be said; except that, in the former, the reins are to be taken in the right hand, and transferred to the left as soon as the seat is reached.

THE SEAT.

The driver should sit in the middle of the box, quite straight towards his horses, rather upright or backward, than forward, with his knees nearly straight, and with his feet together, toward the edge of the footboard. With the exception of a pliant motion of his loins, or any jolting of the coach, his body should be quite at rest, and particularly so when he hits a horse. Independently of appearance, a firm seat on a box is very necessary for safety to a coachman and his passengers, for a trifle will otherwise displace him.

STARTING.

Before starting, four horses should stand clear, or at their proper length from each other. They should have some notice—a click, or a whistle given them to move. If the whip is used, the wheelers should be touched, as generally the ablest horses.

It is with coach-horses as with mankind—that where the physical strength is in the governed, they must be humored a little. When starting, the coachman must not pull at their heads, but feel their mouths lightly, or they may bolt, throw themselves down, or break through their harness. If they are old, and the stage commences with a descent, they should be allowed to go a couple of hundred yards before they are put to their usual pace. A young horse should be started very quietly, making the old horse take collar first. This is especially necessary if the young one is inclined to be hot, as it will prevent his plunging.

A young horse should first be started in a wide space, so that he may be got off without a check. If he be alarmed and inclined to bounce, he should not be held hard, and still less stopped; for, if so, he may not like, particularly if high mettled, to start again. The old horse will prevent his running far. If a young horse be shy of his collar, he should not at first be pressed to it; as he may thereby take a dislike to it, and become a jibber.

A young horse, when first put to a coach, should be turned to the pole very carefully, to prevent its touching his hind quarter, which might make him kick. When he has been driven long enough to be steady, he should be taken up in his bearing-rein, put down lower on his bit, and driven in a wide circle, or figure eight—keeping the inner horse well up to his collar and bit. In breaking, he should be frequently stopped, but not held after being pulled up, as, if high mettled, it will make him restless, and if dull, he does not require it. If, on the contrary, a young horse is heavy, and not ready to start when the command is given, he should be whipped till he answer it.

THE PACES.

These, in driving, must always be a walk or a trot—never a canter, which, owing to the draught, would be equally injurious to the horse and to the carriage. Either of these paces, moreover, should be suited to the nature of the road. Rapid driving, on the stones especially, exposes a carriage to injury, both from shocks against others, and from those which attend its own motion. However, it is sometimes for a moment necessary, in order to get out of the way of carts, wagons, &c.

In public coaches the pace is often too rapid; and, should any passenger plead for the horses, on the score of the excessive heat, the coachman with the utmost *sang froid* replies, that he must keep his time, although the probability sometimes is, that one or more of them may drop, by which considerable time may be lost, as well as reduction in force ensue for the rest of the stage. Horses should be more frequently watered during hot weather than they generally are; increased perspiration renders it necessary.

However well pleased thoughtless people may be in going at an accelerated rate, it is certainly hard that other passengers should be obliged to hazard their existence at the pleasure of a reckless driver, who, in answer to all remonstrance, coolly answers, he must "keep his time." Something should certainly be done to prevent the cantering system;* for no coach, be it ever so well built, can preserve its equilibrium so well when the horses are in the canter or gallop, as when in the trot. At the same time, it is to be borne in mind, that, at the rate our coaches now travel, some slight degree of it may sometimes be unavoidable, owing to horses trotting so variably, and its being very difficult to obtain teams every individual of which shall be able to trot through the distance at the required rate.

In driving four-in-hand, it is not every man who knows when a coach-horse is at work, as a horse may keep a tight

* There is an act which requires that all four shall not gallop together; and many teams, especially in the neighborhood of town, have one good trotter to defeat the informer, known as the "Act of Parliament horse."—ED. Fifth Edition.

trace, and yet be doing little. There is, however, an increased tension of the horse's frame when taking weight with him, which is the surest test, and which never escapes a quick and experienced eye. As already observed, those called lobbing-goers take greater weight with them than horses of finer action, provided they are equally close workers. Heavy draught shortens the stride of horses, after they have been a few years at work.

THE TIME.

In short distances, to know precisely at what time it is necessary to start, to arrive at any place at a certain hour, the driver has only to ascertain the distance, and to regulate the pace by the following table :—

4 miles an hour,	1	mile in	15	minutes.
5	do.	1	do.	12	do.
6	do.	1	do.	10	do.
7	do.	1	do.	$8\frac{1}{2}$	do.
8	do.	1	do.	$7\frac{1}{2}$	do.
9	do.	1	do.	$6\frac{1}{2}$	do.
10	do.	1	do.	6	do.

In the streets of London, ten minutes at least, in every hour must be allowed for stoppages.

THE WHIP.

"We are too apt," said the late Lord Erskine, "to consider animals under the domination of man in no view but that of property. We should never forget that the animal over which we exercise our power has all the organs which render it susceptible of pleasure and pain. It sees, it hears, it smells, it tastes, it feels with acuteness. How mercifully, then, ought we to exercise the dominion entrusted to our care!"

Speaking to coach-horses from the box is now considered slow, but it is not without its effect. Whipping, however, is sometimes indispensable. The manufacture of four-horse whips has arrived at great perfection, and affords employment to many hundred hands.

Refined management of the whip is not of many years' birth; and even now there are but few who execute this effectually and with grace. There are as many ways of whipping coach-horses, says a clever writer in the *Sporting Magazine*, as there are horses in the coach; and, as there is a right and a wrong way of doing most things, a young beginner may observe the following directions, beginning with the wheel-horses :—

Before a coachman hits a wheel-horse, he should twist his thong three times round the crop of his whip, holding the crop at that moment somewhat horizontally, by which means the thong will twist towards the thin end of the crop, when the thong, being doubled, will not exceed the length of a pair-horse thong, and in some measure resemble it. Being double renders it of course more severe, as it falls more heavily on the horse; and by the two ends of the thong not being spread, but close together at the time of the blow, it falls with increased force.

When the off-side wheeler is struck, the coachman's right arm should be put out from his body in the same position in which he presents it to his tailor to measure him for a coat, but the blow should proceed entirely from the wrist. The part on which the horse should be struck is about four inches behind his false belly-band, or somewhere near the short rib on his right side. The stinging part of the blow is then felt under the belly; and, unless he is quite beaten, or of a sulky and bad disposition, he seldom fails to answer it. If he do not answer it here, he must be struck before the belly-band, when the blow falls just behind the fore-arm, on a part on which the skin is very thin. In hitting a near-wheeler, the coachman brings his right hand exactly opposite to his face, and, turning the crop three times around, as before directed, he lets the thong fall sharply across the horse's loins three times in succession, if he do not answer sooner,—observing that, after the third blow, he draws the thong obliquely across the horse's back, by which means his arm returns to a state of rest, and the crop falls gently across his reins, just about his left hand, the crop pointing a little upwards, to prevent the thong getting under or touching the wheel-horse's tail. Should the latter be the case, if the driver lower his crop, the thong will almost always get released; but should it not, he must let the thong loose, and draw it out from the point. When it comes up from the tail, let the coachman throw back his crop a little to his right hand, and the point of the thong will fall across his fingers, when he catches it, and puts it back into his hand. It must be observed, that, in striking the near wheel horse, the wrist only, as in sword exercise, is at work: the body must be quite at rest; and, after the whip is brought to bear, the arm must be quiet also, until the third blow is struck.

There is only one other method of hitting a wheel horse, which is called pointing him. This is done by hitting him with the point of the thong, when loose, just behind his shoulders, but it is not considered neat execution. If there should be a free leader before the bars, it causes him to fret, and is only to be had recourse to in emergencies—as, for instance, in turning round a corner, or into a gate-way, when a leader is to be hit, and before the coachman can recover his thong a wheel horse requires whipping also.

If a wheel horse show symptoms of vice, as a disposition to kick, &c., or, in short, if he refuse to answer either of the other calls upon his exertions, a blow with the double thong on his ears generally brings him to his senses. Without great necessity, however, it is very reprehensible to strike a coach horse over the ears, the parts being very sensible.

It is generally supposed it is in whipping a leader that neatness of execution is more especially displayed. It is, however, quite a mistake to suppose that it is in the power of a coachman to punish a leader with the single, as he can a wheel horse with the double thong. No doubt, however, the blow from the loose thong falls very sharp, as it falls on a tender part, the inside of the thigh.

As the off leader presents himself more fully to the right hand of the coachman than his partner does, the horse that is the less free of the two is generally put on that side. There are but two ways of hitting an off leader: one, by letting the thong fall gently over his neck, or just behind his pad, when his driver merely wishes to refresh his memory, and let him know that he has a whip in his hand; and the other, when he wants to hit him sharply, by striking him with the point of the thong just under his bar. The hard hitters of the old school never conceived they had done the latter effectually, unless they struck their horse twice at least, if not three times, the last stroke always ending in a draw.

As this word "draw" is peculiar to the road, it must be explained to such as may not exactly comprehend it. Suppose a coachman to hit his off leader three times. The first two blows are given, as it were, under-handed, that is to say, the hand is lowered so as to admit of the thong going under the bar the first two strokes. When the third or last is given, the point of the elbow is thrown outwards, so as to incline the thong inwards, which brings it up to the coachman's hand after the stroke, it generally falling across his breast, which would not be the case were it not for the draw. Another advantage also attends the draw: a thong so thrown very seldom hangs in the bars, and nothing is more uncoachman-like than to hit a leader above his bar. A horse's mouth should always be felt before his coachman hits him.

Hitting the near leader with neatness and effect is the most difficult part of the use of the whip. There are two ways of doing it: one, by two common strokes and the draw; and the other by a sort of back-handed stroke, which is a very neat one, and sufficiently severe, but it does not bring the thong so immediately up to the coachman's hand as the drawn stroke does. In the back-handed stroke, the wrist describes an exact figure of eight, and the arm cannot be kept, as before, quite still. In the other method of hitting, the coachman's arm is brought about opposite his chin, the first two blows proceeding from the wrist alone; but in the third, or the draw, the hand descends, the elbow is thrown outwards, and by two jerks of the arm, which it is difficult to describe on paper, the draw is effected, and the thong comes, as before stated, across the coachman's breast, so as to enable him to catch it instantly.

There is one other way of hitting a leader; and that is, by what is called the chop. This is done by throwing out the right arm rather forward, and with it, of course, the thong, and then bringing it back sharply with the wrist inclined downwards. The thong falls severely on the horse's thigh, and comes up to the hand again, as in the draw. This is a very useful blow in a narrow confined place, or when it is necessary to lose no time before a leader is hit; and, when neatly done, has a very workman-like appearance. This blow generally falls above the bar, particularly if a horse is not at work at the time.

It has been said that leaders should always be hit under their bar. This, however, cannot always be done; for if a horse hang back from his collar, his bar is so low that it may be difficult to get under it. In this case, however, the blow is made to tell smartly, as it is in the coachman's power to throw his whip into the flank, which is a very sensible part. When a leader is well up to his collar, he always can, and always should, be hit under his bar.

Should the point of the thong catch, or, as they say on the road, "get hanged," in the bars or the pole-pieces—neither of which it will do when properly drawn after the last stroke, as the inclination of the hand in the act of drawing enables it to clear them—no violence should be used to loosen it, or a broken crop will be the consequence. On the contrary, the arm should be thrown forward, and the thong lightly moved, when in a minute or two it will shake out. If it be fast between the eye of the main bar and the pole-hook, the leaders should be eased a little, and it will get released. Sometimes, however, on a wet day, a thong will lap round some of these things so fast as to make it necessary for the guard or some person to get down to untie it. This is technically called having a bite. The double thong will also sometimes hitch in the ends of the wheelers' traces, as also in the point of the false belly-band. To obviate this, in gentlemen's harness, these parts are always covered, or piped, as it is called.

A free leader should not be hit in a short turn, or he may break his bar, perhaps the pole-hook, or even the main bar. Neither should leaders be hit in going over a small bridge which is much raised, or when the pole points upwards, as their draught on the end of it may snap it in the futchels. Some drivers perpetually whip or fan their horses, which first irritates and afterwards injures them, by rendering them insensible to the proper aids or correction. It must be observed that the whip should never be used but in case of necessity. Indeed, one of the best proofs of a good coachman is to see his right arm still; and although, for the safety of his coach, he ought to be able to punish a horse when he requires punishment, yet he should, on all accounts, be as sparing of it as he can. Horses may be whipped till they become callous to whipping, and therefore slow. In the condition in which coach horses are now kept, a pound of Nottingham whipcord will last a good coachman his lifetime. The very act of throwing the point of the thong over the leaders' heads, or letting it fall on their backs, as a fisherman throws his fly upon the stream, will set half the coach horses in England, in these days, into a gallop.

THOROUGHFARES, PASSING, &c.

The driver should avoid passing through the great thoroughfares, and prefer the widest of the less frequented streets which run parallel to them. In London, he should never go into the City through the Strand, Fleet-street, and Cheapside, between twelve and five o'clock, if he can possibly avoid it, as these streets are then crowded with every kind of vehicle. He should also avoid going into the City about mid-day, on Mondays and Fridays, on account of the droves of oxen passing through the principal streets.

The middle of the road is safest, especially for a loaded coach, except under peculiar circumstances.

In driving four horses, to keep them well in hand is a

most material point, both as regards their work and for the safety of the coach. The track made by a coach in descending a hill shows whether the horses are properly held together or not. Accidents from horses taking fright, and bolting across the road, happen only to clumsy fellows, of whom the list is considerable. The rules for passing and meeting carriages on the road have already been given, yet there are times when they need not be strictly adhered to, and a little accommodation becomes expedient. Thus, if one coachman has the hill in his favor—that is, if he be going down, and a loaded coach be coming up at the same time—he who is descending, if he can do it with safety, ought to give the hardest side of the road to the other coachman.

As to narrow spaces, it is evident that where the bars can go the coach can go, as they are wider than the wheels; and consequently, if they are cleared, all is safe. The swing-bar is an excellent invention, as a horse works in it from either shoulder, and therefore quite at his ease. A sharp and experienced driver may calculate exactly the space sufficient to pass between two bodies at rest, and may therefore pass with confidence and at ease. As, however, in streets, he must meet many carriages driven by inexperienced or intoxicated fellows, who do not for a moment move in any direct line, he should allow them ample room, and proceed with the utmost caution. A driver must be incessantly on the look-out, must watch every vehicle that approaches, and give it more room than it may seem to require.

ASCENDING AND DESCENDING.

In going up hill, it is in general best to trot up at first, and to walk afterwards. In going down hill, it is best to

keep the wheelers tight in hand, to let the leaders just
clear the bars, and to come gently down. In the latter
case, a turn of the reins of the wheel-horses may be made
round the little finger. (Plate XLIII. fig. 4.)

Although, however, it may be necessary to catch up
wheel-horses, and make them hold back their coach down
hill, there is nothing in which a light finger is more essential to safety. The manner in which some persons haul at
horses' mouths, when descending with a load, considerably
adds to the difficulty, by trying the strength of the tackle.
But this is not all: these persons should be aware that all
this force employed on their horses' mouths is so much
added to the pressure of the coach; in proportion to it is
that pressure increased. The horses are then drawing by
their heads!

The objection to a locked wheel, with a top-heavy load,
have already been stated. If, however, with a heavy load,
and upon a smooth hard road, a wheel must be locked, it
should be that next a ditch, or other dangerous part. In
going down hill, a coach always strikes on the side on which
the wheel is not locked. The coachman should therefore
keep as much as possible on that side of the road on which
the wheel is locked: by crossing the road, if he meet or
have to pass any thing, the coach will not strike; and by
holding that way, at any time, it will prevent overturning.
The coach naturally strikes in a direct line from the perch-
bolt.

The generality of passengers know not the danger of galloping a coach, with three tons' weight in and out, down
hill, at the rate of twelve or fifteen miles an hour, with no
wheel locked, the whole resistance of the wheel-horses depending on a small leather strap and buckle at the top of
the hames,—these coachmen deeming it beneath their

Plate XLIV

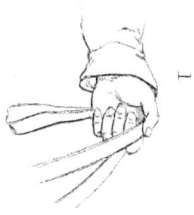

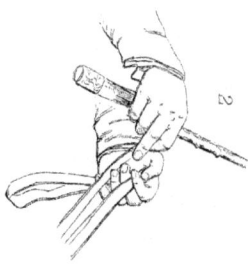

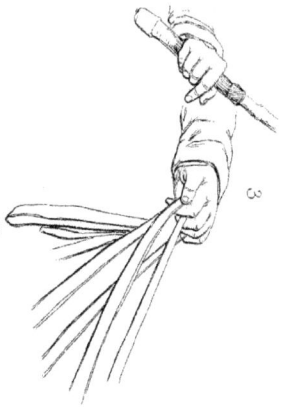

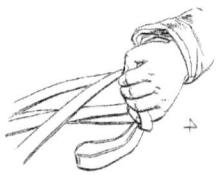

The Rein-hold in Driving

dignity to drive with breechings. Even thus, however, accidents would be much less frequent if coachmen took the precaution of pulling up their horses short, when on the point of descending. In night-work, this is doubly useful, because it often happens that a pole-chain is unhooked, or a hame-strap gets loose, without being discernible by lamp or moonlight.

"With wheel-horses that will hold back at all, I will be bound," says a clever writer and experienced coachman, "to take a loaded coach down most of the hills now met with on our great roads, without a drag-chain, provided I am allowed to pull up my horses at the top, and let them take it quietly the first hundred yards. This, it may be said, would be losing time, but, on the contrary, time would be gained by it; for, as soon as I perceived I was master of my coach, I should let her go, and by letting my horses loose at the bottom, I could spring them into a gallop, and cheat them out of half the hill, if there were one (as frequently happens) on the next portion of the road. This advantage, it must be recollected, cannot be taken if the chain be to be put on; and I have therefore in my favor all the time required to put the chain on, and to take it off again."

There are, however, some horses which no man can make to hold a loaded coach down hill. Of this description are, first, the stiff-necked one, as he is called, who turns his head away from his partner, and shoulders the pole; and, secondly, one who, when he feels the weight pressing upon him, begins to canter and jump, as coachmen term it; with these holding back properly is out of the question. With such cattle, the drag-chain must be had recourse to; as well as when there is the least reason to suspect the soundness of the harness. All this confirms the necessity of checking the force of a coach before descending a steep hill, and, indeed, in some cases—as with bad holders—before coming upon a slight descent. The term which coachmen have for this species of road, is "pushing ground;" and if the fall be long, it is astonishing how the pressure of a loaded coach upon wheel horses is increased before getting to the bottom of it, and how difficult it would be, with wheelers not of the very best stamp, to pull up short, if any accident should happen.

Young coachmen, in descending a hill, should take care that their leaders do not draw on the end of the pole, which many free ones do when they find the coach coming quickly after them; for this not only increases the pressure of the coach on the wheelers, but, should either of them stumble, it must assist in bringing him down. The following good and characteristic directions were given by a very experienced coachman, to a gentleman who undertook to take his coach a journey for him, but who, although he knew the road well, had never driven on it before. "That middle twelve miles of ground," said he, "is a punisher, and you must mind what you are at with this load. You have two hills to go down, and three to go up, in the first seven miles. Don't stop to put the chain on, as they'll hold well, and the tackle is good; and don't let them walk up the hills, for they are bad hands at that—you will lose a horse's draught by it, and perhaps get hung up on one of them. You must take fifty minutes to do the first seven miles, and good work too. When you get at the top of the last hill, get down and put your near leader to the cheek, and they'll toddle you over the last five miles in half an hour, with all the pleasure alive."

The following observations on this subject from the number of the *Quarterly Review* already quoted, are too interesting to be omitted here.

" Many years have elapsed," he says, " since I first observed that, somehow or other, the horses on the continent
manage to pull a heavy carriage up a steep hill, or even
along a dead level, with greater ease to themselves than our
English horses. If any unprejudiced person would only
attentively remark with what little apparent fatigue three
small ill-conditioned horses will draw, not only his own carriage, but very often that huge overgrown vehicle the
French diligence, or the German eilwagen, I think he
would agree with me; but the whole equipment is so un-
sightly—the rope harness is so rude—the horses without
blinkers look so wild—there is so much bluster with the
postilion—that, far from paying any compliment to the turn-
out, one is very much disposed at once to condemn the
whole thing, and, not caring a straw whether such horses
be fatigued or not, to make no other remark than that in
England one would have travelled at nearly twice the rate
with one-tenth of the noise. But neither the rate nor the
noise is the point—our superiority in the former, and our
inferiority in the latter, cannot be doubted. The thing to
account for is, how such small, weak horses do actually
manage to draw a heavy carriage up hill with so much ease
to themselves. Now, in English, French, and German
harness, there exists, as it were, three degrees of comparison
as to the manner in which the head of the horse is treated;
for, in England, it is elevated, or borne up, by what we
call the bearing-rein,—in France it is left as nature placed
it (there being to common French harness no bearing-rein,)
—and, in Germany, the head is tied down to the lower
extremity of the collar, or else the collar is so made that
the animal is by it deprived of the power of raising his
head. Now, passing over for a moment the French method,
which is, in fact, the state of nature, let us for a moment

22*

consider which is better—to bear a horse's head up, as in England, or to pull it downwards, as in Germany."

Evidently fired with a favorite theme, he thus proceeds:—
"In a state of nature, the wild horse, as every body knows (?) has two distinct gaits or attitudes. If man, or any still wilder beast, come suddenly upon him, up goes his head; and as he first stalks and then trots gently away —with ears erect, snorting with his nose, and proudly snuffing up the air, as if exulting in his freedom—as one fore-leg darts before the other, we have before us a picture of doubt, astonishment, and hesitation, all of which feelings seem to rein him, like a troop-horse, on his haunches; but, attempt to pursue him, and the moment he defiés you —the moment, determining to escape, he shakes his head, and lays himself to his work—how completely does he alter his attitude ! That instant down goes his head, and from his ears to the tip of his tail there is in his vertebræ an undulating action which seems to propel him, which works him along, and which, it is evident, you could not deprive him of without materially diminishing his speed. Now, in harness, the horse has naturally the same two gaits or attitudes, and it is quite true that he can start away with a carriage either in the one or the other; but the means by which he succeeds in this effort—the physical powers which he calls into action, are essentially different: in the one case he works by his muscles, and in the other by his own dead, or rather living weight. In order to grind corn, if any man were to erect a steam-engine over a fine, strong, running stream, we should all say to him, 'Why do you not allow your wheel to be turned by cold water instead of hot ? Why do you not avail yourself of the weight of the water, instead of expending your capital in converting it into the power of steam ? In short, why

do you not use the simple resource which Nature has presented ready-made to your hand ?'   In the same way, the
German might say to us, ' We acknowledge a horse can
drag a carriage by the power of his muscles, but why do
you not allow him to drag it by his weight ?'

"Let any one observe a pair of English post-horses dragging a heavy weight up a hill, and he will at once see that
the poor creatures are working by their muscles, and that
it is by sheer strength that the resistance is overcome : but
how can it be otherwise; their heads are higher than nature
intended them to be, even in walking in a state of liberty,
carrying no weight but themselves: the balance of their
bodies is therefore absolutely turned against, instead of
leaning in favor of their draught; and if my reader will
pass his hands down the back sinews of our stage-coach or
post-chaise horses, he will soon feel (though not so keenly
as they do,) what is the cruel and fatal consequence.   It is
true, that in ascending a very steep hill an English
postilion will occasionally unhook his bearing-reins; but the
jaded creatures, trained for years to work in a false attitude, cannot in one moment get themselves into the scientific position which the German horses are habitually
encouraged to adopt.   Besides this, we are so sharp with
our horses,—we keep them so constantly on the *qui vive*, or,
as wĕ term it, in hand, that we are always driving them from
the use of their weight to the application of their sinews.
That the figure and attitude of a horse working by his
sinews are infinitely prouder than when he is working by
his weight, (there may exist, however, false pride among
horses as well as men,) I most readily admit; and therefore, for carriages of luxury, where the weight bears little
proportion to the powers of the noble animals employed, I
acknowledge that the sinews are more than sufficient ; but,

to bear up the head of a poor horse at plough, or at any slow, heavy work, is, I conceive, a barbarous error, which ought not to be persisted in.

"Whether there is most of a horse in a German, or of the German in a horse, is a nice point, on which people might argue a great deal; but the broad fact really is, that Germans live on more amicable terms with their horses, and understand their dispositions infinitely better, than the English; in short, they treat them as horses, while we act towards them and drill them as if they were men; and, in case any reader should doubt that Germans are better horse masters than we are, I beg to remind him of what is perfectly well known to the British army,—namely, that in the Peninsular war the cavalry horses of the German Legion was absolutely fat, while those of our regiments were skin and bone."

THE TURNINGS.

These must be regulated by the ground. A good driver avoids all quick and sharp turnings. In town, it is much better to drive on a little further, where another street may allow the ample room requisite in turning. If a carriage do not pass quite across a channel without turning, the perch must be twisted according to the descent, because one wheel falls as that at the opposite angle rises. By such a wrench, especially when going fast, the main or perch bolt is frequently broken, and every part strained.

A loaded coach should never be turned short, even at a slow pace, for the coach is never safe when there is not an even bearing on the transom beds. If turned short, at a quick pace, the higher and looser part of a coach must go over, because all bodies put in motion by one power will proceed in a straight line, unless compelled to change their course by some force impressed. Hence a horse at full speed is with difficulty turned to right or left; and, if he turn suddenly, and of his own accord, he puts his rider's horsemanship to the test. So with a coach, a sudden turn to one side the road allows the body to swag towards the other, and the centre of gravity is lost.

In a turn, a coachman must point his leaders well, that is, take proper ground for them to make the turn, and let his wheelers follow them. Moreover, as wheel-horses are always in haste to make the turn, the driver must shoot them out on the opposite side, just as he has pointed his leaders. Thus, if the turn be to the right, he must catch up his near wheel rein, and hit his off-wheel horse; and *vice versâ*. This will keep the head of the pole (which he should have his eye upon) just between the leaders, and the wheelers will follow, as if they were running on a straight road. This will also secure him against danger, by clearing his coach of posts, gutters, &c. No man can make a neat turn with four horses, unless he shoot his wheelers, at the same time that he points his leaders. In turning, the wheelers must rather be kept up, and the leaders be tight in hand, to avoid the corner; for, if the wheelers flag, and the leaders draw, the carriage must be brought against it.

THE RANKS IN TOWN.

These must never be broken, either in driving through crowded streets, or in setting down at crowded places. As to admitting others into the rank, every driver should do as he would be done by.

STOPS.

It is a good plan to use horses to stop by notice, as it may prevent accidents. In pulling up, the driver must pull the reins equally, but rather those of the wheelers first. If this is attended with difficulty, take the wheelers' reins in the right hand, and pull till they hang well on the breeching, or on the pole chains, thus increasing the leaders' draught so much that they will easily be pulled up.

When a young coach horse is stopped, it should be very gradually—allowing at least ten yards to do it in; for, if it be attempted to stop him short, he will resist. A careful driver will never keep his carriage standing in a great thoroughfare; but when obliged to stop in a crowded street, the driver should, if possible, avoid the spot where another carriage is stopping; should choose as much as possible the widest part of the street; and draw up close to the curb.

There is no part of stage-coach economy in which greater alteration has been made than in changing horses. Unless business is to be transacted—as taking fares for passengers, setting down, getting out parcels, &c.,—the average with fast coaches is three minutes for each change.

ACCIDENTS, ETC. TO HORSES.

A cantering leader, or one that frets, is generally mismanaged by young coachmen. They are apt to pull him back, and endeavor to get him to trot, by the bit, which generally fails, or makes him even worse, by bringing him back on his bar. The right way is to pull him back by his harness; that is, to keep the wheelers back, so that he may feel his collar and bit at the same time.

A horse that kicks ought to be taken very short in his pole-piece, and gagged; and, when he begins to kick, he should be whipped on the ears—a punishment which should never be inflicted but for vice. Hallooing to a horse when he kicks, has sometimes an effect. A hot leader is sometimes benefited by mopping. An experienced driver says, "I once bought a capital coach horse for twenty-six pounds, because no one could drive him; and as he had broken two carriages, he was the terror of the neighborhood. I mopped him, and could drive him with the greatest safety, either leader or at wheel."

In the case of a horse falling, a periodical writer, replying to another, states, "In one of his letters on 'The Road,' he says, 'If the coachman be driving with the short wheel rein, and a horse fall beyond recovery, he had better open his hand, and let the reins fall out, than run the risk of being pulled off the box.' With all due deference to such authority, I cannot subscribe to this, as it frequently happens that a horse falls, is dragged along the ground for a short distance, and recovers himself the moment the coach stops, and then starts off at full gallop, the other horses following his example. Now, if coachee has opened his fist, and let the reins tumble out, and the above occurrence should take place, I would certainly rather be on the top of Cheviot than on the top of the said coach, as the catastrophe would not be very difficult to foretell."

On many horses, hot weather has a singular effect; and, therefore, it often happens that a good winter horse is an indifferent summer one. Coach horses are subject to many accidents, of which one is peculiar to them—namely, fracture of the legs in trotting on level ground.* Fractures

* When driving one of the Birmingham fast coaches, just entering the town of Dunstable, my near leader fell with her off hind leg snapped clean in two, held together merely by the skin. On pulling up to clear her from the coach, I found the cause of the accident; a piece of flint, shaped like a hatchet, and with a blade as keen as a razor, still adhering to the bone, against which it had either been whirled by a kick from one of the other three, or had flown upwards from the tread of the mare herself.—ED. Fifth Edition.

of the foot in draught-horses and others are common; but fractures of the leg in coach-horses when trotting over level ground, are probably caused by over-tension of the limb in the act of drawing. It is said that a coach horse's leg is more frequently broken, when, with a heavy load behind him, he snatches at his collar in a turn of the road.

They are also subject to an affection known by the appellation of the lick, which greatly injures their condition. In this state they lick each other's skins, and gnaw their halters 'to pieces. This probably proceeds from the state of the stomach, caused by the excitement of high feeding and work. It may be removed by opening or alterative medicines.

They are likewise subject to a kind of vertigo, which on the road is called megrims. This, of which the immediate cause is temporary pressure on the brain, is often brought on by running in the face of a hot sun; and, therefore, horses subject to megrims ought to work at night. The attack appears to come on suddenly, though a snatching motion of the head is sometimes observed to precede it. If not immediately pulled up, the horse thus affected drops. Such horses should have attention paid to the state of their bowels, and have frequent antimonial alteratives. What is called " a megrim horse" is always dangerous, especially near a precipice or ditch, as, when seized, he rolls away from his partner, and, of course, takes him with him.

ACCIDENTS TO COACHES, ETC.

A necessary precaution in a gig is—never to sit with the feet under the body, but always to have one, if not both, out before it. " I had a passenger by the side of me," says the driver who gives this caution, "who was

sitting with his feet under his belly, and who was consequently thrown with much violence into the road. I had
five miles further to drive him, during which he took care
to have his feet before him."

In stage-coaches, accidents no doubt occur, and no one
will assert that the proprietors guard against them to the
utmost of their power. The great competition, however,
which*they have to encounter, is a strong stimulant to
their exertions on this score. In some respects, also, the
increase of pace has become the traveller's security:
coaches and harness must be of the best quality; horses
fresh and sound; coachmen of skill and respectability can
alone be employed; and to this increased pace is owing
the improvement in these men's character. They have
not time now for drinking, and they come in collision with
a class of persons superior to those who formerly were
stage-coach passengers, by whose example it has been
impossible for them not to profit. A coachman drunk on
his box is now a rarity—a coachman quite sober was, but
a few years ago, still more so. On the whole, however,
travelling by public conveyance was never so secure as it
is at the present time. Axle-trees and springs do not often
break now; and if proprietors go to the expense, their
wheels are made secure against coming off.

The worst accidents, and those which, with the present
structure of coaches, can never be entirely provided against,
arise from broken axle-trees, and wheels coming off on the
road. The guard, therefore, in whose department this
lies, ought to examine the axle tree every time it is fresh
greased. He should also remove it once in ten days, put
a string through the bolt that receives the linch-pin, and
hang it up and cleanse it; and he should then strike it
with a hammer, when, if uncracked and sound, it will ring

23

like a bell—the coachman attending to take care that it be again properly screwed on.

Reins also break, though rarely, except in those parts which run through the terrets, the rings of the throat-lash, or in the billets; and attention to these would make all safe, as far as accidents from this cause are concerned.

Accidents happen also from want of attention to the security of the bridles. The throat-lash, therefore—particularly of the wheelers—should be as tight as can be allowed without injuring respiration. There otherwise is always danger of the bridle being pulled off. Accidents, moreover, happen from galloping coach horses down hill, or on even ground. If, indeed, a casualty then happen, it must be a bad one. The goodness of a road is no preservative against it; on the contrary, it is possible that if a coach begin to swing, it may go over from the very circumstance of the road being so level and so smooth that there is nothing on its surface to hold the wheels to the ground. If, moreover, there be two horses at wheel whose stride in their gallop differs much as to extent, the unequal draught invariably sets the coach rolling, and, unless the pace moderate, the fore-wheel passing over even a small stone, may, under such circumstances, cause the coach to upset. In respect to lateral motion, however, much depends upon the build of the carriage. In galloping coach-horses, if the leaders lead off with two legs, the motion of the coach is considerably truer, and the swing-bars are also much more at rest, than when each horse uses the same leg.

It appears, then, that accidents to coaches are chiefly to be attributed either to the want of proper skill and care in the servants employed, or to what is still less pardonable, inattention on the part of their masters. Road-coachmen, fortunately, are well aware that the law looks sharply after them; and that for neglect proved against them, they are equally answerable to their employers, as these are to the public.

"If I were to go upon the road," says an amateur, "I would be a night coachman through a well-inhabited country. For six months of the year it is undoubtedly the pleasanter service; and I never found any difference between taking rest by day or by night." It is, however, calculated only for a man in the prime of his days, as all his energies are required. The night coachman ought to know his line of road well. He must take rest regularly, or he will be sure to become drowsy, if he do not go to sleep. He must also keep himself sober; keep a tight hand on his horses; keep the middle of the road; and be sure to keep time.

The night coachman must cast his eye well forward, and get out of the way of carts and wagons in time. Although, by looking perpendicularly from his box or at the hedges, if there be any, he may always see if he be in the road; yet, if he cannot throw his eye some way before his leaders' heads, he is going at random. He will often get close to things he may meet in the road before he is aware of them; and, therefore, as I have already said, it is essential that he should be wide awake, and have his horses well in hand.

Chains and springs on the bars are good things for night-work, as they prevent the leaders' traces coming off. A narrow road, sufficiently wide, of course, for carriages to pass with convenience—with no ditch on the side—is much the best for night-work. Unless when the moon is very bright, a dark night is in favor of safe travelling. When it is what coachmen term "a clear dark," the lamps give much better light than when the darkness approaches to grey.

In very wide roads, particularly where there are no hedges to confine them, lamplight is both weak and deceiving; and moonlight is often glimmering and doubtful, particularly when clouds are passing rapidly. Lamplight is treacherous, both in fogs and when horses are going at a moderate pace, with the wind just behind them; for then the steam arising from their bodies follows them, and necessarily obstructs the light. Sometimes, from driven rain or snow, a coachman can scarcely open his eyes so as to see the road to the extent of the light given by the lamps; in which case a tight hand on the horses is especially necessary.

A heavy fog is the only thing which baffles the skill and intrepidity of our night coachmen. In this case, lamps are of no avail as to showing light forward; and, in the worst cases, the only use that can be made of them is, for the guard to hold one in his hand behind the coach, by which he will be able to see whether the horses are in the road or not. Lamps, however, are always useful in the case of accidents; and, except in very clear moonlight, a night coach should never travel without them.

Accidents often occur from coachmen neglecting to light their lamps in going into a town. It often happens that, when a coach comes down the road in the morning, there may be no obstruction in the streets; but rubbish from buildings, stones, or many other things, may be thrown out by the time it comes up again at night. When an accident happens to a coach, presence of mind is much required. Outside passengers should never think of quitting by jumping, from the fore part, a least, until she falls to the ground. From the box, indeed, a man may get over the roof into the guard's seat, and thence descend.

Among the various contrivances for dragging wheels, we may mention a very ingenious one by Mr. Rapson. The drag is applied to the nave of the wheel, with a chain attached, which is fastened to the breeching, a small pin on each side going into the bar of the drag. If one of these pins be taken out, the wheel will be dragged, and if both are withdrawn, the wheels are both acted upon during the descent, by the breech bearing against the horse.

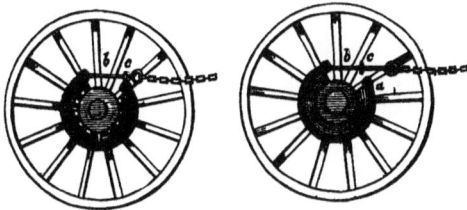

In the first of these diagrams we have a representation of the break attached to the wheel, but inoperative, the jointed circle separating the chain, c, and bolt, b, from the nave. In the second figure, the entire frame, a, b, c, is seen in direct collision with the nave, and by its friction retarding the locked wheel. This, however, does not occur till the breeching of the harness is drawn tight by the pressure of the carriage upon it.

OBSTRUCTIONS, OFFENCES, AND INJURIES.

By the 1st Geo. I. c. 57, drivers of hackney coaches are to give way to gentlemen's carriages, under a penalty of 10s.

If a carriage be obstructed by disorderly persons, the driver should take out his pocket-book, and let the persons guilty of this see that he is taking a note of their number; and he should then coolly tell them that he will summon them if they do not immediately clear the way.

If a carriage be injured by another running against it,

the driver should ascertain whose carriage has done the mischief, and let his coachmaker give an estimate of the charge for repairing it; but, before he has it done, he should let the person who injured it see the mischief, and pay the charge; or, as is the custom, let the repair be made by the coachmaker of the party who committed the injury.

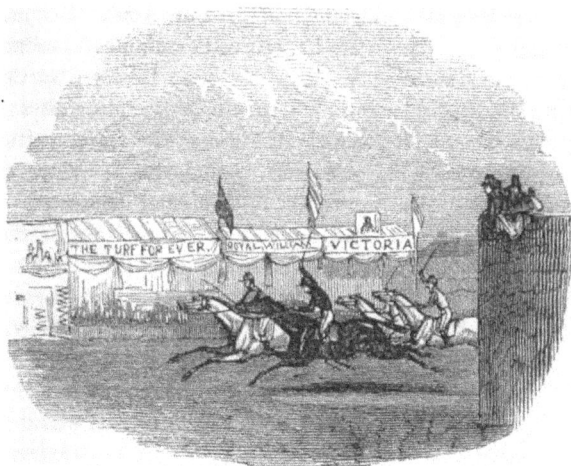

THE TURF.

It is singular that no portion of our domestic annals should be so obscure as that which relates to the early history of our first of National Sports. In the remotest ages of civilization (so far at least as any existing records carry us back,) a taste for horse-racing was fostered and promoted as a social engine peculiarly adapted to rural and political purposes. The Greeks—the wisest and most polished people that the world has ever seen—carried their estimate of its importance so far, that their chiefs not only took part in the sports of the hippodrome, but acted as officials in the regulation of its details. Philip of Macedon thought it not unbecoming the imperial crown, that he who wore it should discharge the office of judge at the Pythian Games, and his son repaid in gold every line written by Pindar in honor of the chaplet of wild olive.* The verse of Pindar, and the

* The crown given to the victors in the Olympic games.

prose of Pausanias, have immortalized the names of Olympia and Elis. The latter has left us the minutest particulars of the economy of racing in his day. He describes the Olympian Hippodrome at Elis, and all its gorgeous display of splendid embellishments and ingenious machinery, with a care and prodigality of narrative that give assurance of the importance which attached to the matter delineated.— Of the perfection to which, in that era, the science of the course had attained, we need no better proof than the classification observed in the Olympic Games—where horses were matched according to their ages, and prizes instituted for races between mares only (called Calpe.) It is needless, however, to encumber our subject with ancient lore, by continuing these classic references. Enough has, perhaps, been already adduced to establish this point—that we possess more knowledge of the condition of racing three thousand years ago, than we do of the state it was in three hundred years since in our native land.

But because we are in possession of such scanty materials, it by no means follows that the little we do know should be withheld. The reader will therefore have the courtesy to look back with me to the tenth century, and I promise to bring him again into the nineteenth with all convenient speed. As far back, then, as the reign of Athelstan (925,) we read that a present of " running horses" was sent to that monarch from France, the gift of Hugh Capet. As nothing however is known of the character of those animals, we will pass on to the reign of William, which affords better data. At that period a nobleman (the Earl of Shrewsbury) appears to have imported several Spanish horses for his own use. Now, as the Moors had had a footing in Spain for several centuries prior to the Norman conquest, there is little doubt that the blood of the Barb was, in the eleventh century, extensively diffused through that country, and that a highly improved breed of the horse was at the time extant there. Here we have a reasonable era from which to date an amelioration of the indigenous race in our island. A little more than a century later, in the reign of Henry the Second (1154,) we come to, as far as I have been able to discover, the earliest mention of racing to be found in our national records. This refers to a barbarous sort of running practised upon the plain now occupied by Smithfield, which does not appear to have been subjected to any regulations of time or method. Smithfield, indeed, was then the great horse-mart, and very probably the contests, exalted by their chronicler (Fitzstephen the monk,) to Olympic honors, were nothing more than exhibitions, by rival horse-croupers, of the mettle, speed, and action of their respective "palfreys, hackneys, and charging steeds."

Still, that horse-racing was about this time a popular pastime, and one in which the nobles of the land were wont to take pride, is fully established by the allusions to it that abound in the many metrical legends, yet in existence, composed in honor of Richard of the Lion Heart. These preserve the names of the coursers, and speak of them as being valued at sums that, allowing for the difference in the worth of money, quite exceed any prices known in our day. The domestic troubles which marked the reign of John, and the succession of wars in which we were subsequently engaged, probably interrupted the progress of this sport materially—at all events, we do not find any of our sovereigns giving their countenance to it from Richard to the bluff Harry. Henry VIII. was constitutionally disposed for manly occupations and amusements—of his moral tendencies we speak not. We have it on the authority of Challoner that he was much disposed to improve the breed of horses, for which purpose he imported various descriptions from Spain· and Turkey. Fortune, too, enabled his daughter Elizabeth to do much for our native breed; the destruction of the Spanish Armada having supplied us with many barbs and Spanish-bred horses, their descendants, found in the vessels of that fleet which fell into the hands of Lord Howard of Effingham.

We now come to her successor, James I.,* who must be considered as a founder of legitimate racing in this country. He introduced the first Arab into England of which we have any knowledge—that purchased by Mr. Markham, and known as the Markham Arabian. The training system, which has now reached such perfection, was then practised in its various divisions of physic, work, sweating, and the etcetera of stable economy; and the weight to be carried for public prizes arranged by authority. The Roodee, at Chester, was an established course in this reign, one of the prizes being a silver bell, of the value of ten pounds or thereabouts, run for in five-mile heats. Similar prizes were also given at Theobald's on Enfield Chase, at Croydon, and Gatherly, in Yorkshire, whence the popular term "bearing the bell," no doubt, had its origin. His unfortunate son Charles I. had little opportunity of forwarding the social concerns of himself or others. In his reign, however, the first races on record at Newmarket were held, and, by a similar fatality, to Newmarket was he borne a prisoner to the parliamentary forces. The "civil dudgeon" of the Protectorate of course was not friendly to the amusements of the turf, but, though suspended, they were not lost sight of. Mr. Place, the stud-master to Oliver

---

* The palace at Newmarket was built by this monarch for the purpose of enjoying the diversion of hunting—no races having been held upon the heath till the succeeding reign.

Cromwell, imported the celebrated horse known as the White Turk. He was also the owner of some very capital mares, one of which, during the search after Cromwell's property at the Restoration, he saved from destruction by hiding in a vault, whence she took the name of the "Coffin Mare."

With the Restoration came the palmy days of the turf. Regular meetings were established at Newmarket, and various other parts of England; silver cups and bowls of the value of one hundred pounds were presented as royal gifts, and, more than all, the light of royal favor shone upon it in shape of Charles the Debonair and Mistress Eleanor Gwynne. William III. had no taste for racing, and died by a fall from his horse. Prince George of Denmark, on the other hand, was warmly attached to the Turf, and promoted its interest by every means in his power. We are indebted for many royal plates to his influence with his consort Queen Anne. George I. was no sportsman; in his reign, however, the alteration in the royal plates took place, by which a sum of one hundred guineas was substituted in their stead. Shortly after George II. ascended the throne, arose a morbid yearning after legislating for the Turf. Some of the acts enacted were mischievous; very many were very silly; one was good:—"That no plate or prize of a less value than £50 should be run for, under a penalty of £200." It was during this reign that the Darley and Godolphin Arabians were brought into this country,—two horses from whom have descended all the most celebrated racers that adorn the annals of our turf. This is the period at which the genealogy of our unrivalled thorough-bred horse then, was *naturalized*, and it is the date whence I think it most convenient to begin my notice of English racing.

Even a notice so confined as this is beset with obscurities that few would conceive possible. As an instance, I will adduce the case of an old and well-informed inhabitant of Epsom, who some years ago published a very clever history of that place. He starts somewhere about the Conquest, and never halts for want of materials as he goes on, till he comes to the great stumbling-block, concerning which he shall speak for himself:—" When the races on Epsom Downs were first held periodically, *we have not been able to trace;* but we find that from the year 1730 they have been annually held in the months of May or June, and about six weeks previous to which the hunters' stakes are occasionally run for on the Epsom race course, at one of which, in 1730, the famous horse Madcap won the prize, and proved the best plate-horse in England."

To return, however, to the reign of George II., though we find little bearing on the business of the Turf to be gleaned from its records, it introduces us to the great forefathers of our thorough blood, and stirs one of the most interesting questions in our domestic natural history—the problem of the seed or origin of the English thoroughbred horse. A brief search through the stud-book will convince the inquirer that, almost without exception, our great racers were and are descendants of the Darley and Godolphin Arabians : I use the latter term merely because its conventionality now identifies those celebrated animals. They were both, as has been stated, imported in this reign : the question that I would here investigate applies equally to each, but, for the sake of simplifying it, I will treat it with reference to the latter only. "That he was a genuine Arabian," says the stud-book, " his excellence as a sire is deemed sufficient proof;" a little further on we read, " It is remarkable that there is not a *superior* horse now on the

Turf without a cross of the Godolphin Arabian, neither has there been for several years past." The probable date of his arrival in this country was 1725, or thereabouts. Hundreds of Arabs had preceded him as sires, their introduction for that purpose having been a very general speculation from the time of Charles I. That the indigenous island breed had thereby been rendered good service, there can be no doubt; but that the Turf derived any signal advantages from the importations is more than problematical.

Are our celebrated strains of racing blood derived at all from an Arab source, and, if so descended, are they excellent *consequently*, or of accident? As regards the first moiety of the inquiry, a work has just appeared in Paris, the production of a gentleman of some literary celebrity,* relating to the genealogy of the horse so long known to us as the Godolphin Arabian. His statements go to show that he was a pure *Barb*, presented, with seven others, by the Bey of Tunis to Louis XV., *about* the year 1731. All the portraits I have ever seen of him certainly go to strengthen this reading of his descent, and proclaim him not of Asiatic origin. The date is an erroneous one, as he was a sire in England in the year in which he is said to have reached France; but we must be content with very vague data in all that concerns our subject a century ago. As to the second division of the question, after-time must furnish the means of replying to it, if it be ever answered. My bias is to a belief that there exist families of the horse in the East possessed of a perfection infinitely surpassing any generically inherited. This I have attempted to demonstrate in a work upon which I am at present engaged,

* M. Eugene Sue.

24

some portion of which has been already published.* The
fact (of which I was made conscious by authority beyond
question) that the Imaum of Muscat, one of the most
powerful sovereign princes of India, expended ten years of
active search, backed by the enormous bribe of ten thousand
pounds, before he could procure a descendant of a line
sufficiently pure to present to King George IV., seems to
establish the truth of the theory to which I profess being
inclined.   All that we learn from our knowledge of the almost religious veneration with which the genealogy of the
horse is treated in the East, goes to the like confirmation.
"It is remarkable that there is not a *superior* horse *now*
on the Turf without a cross of the Godolphin Arabian."
I leave the reader to interpret as his own reflections may
lead him.

Shall I venture, at the hazard of pursuing my theory
"ultra fines," to offer one more example in support of it?
That no structural organization available to the eye, no individual excellence in the parents, influence, in our raising
stock, the performances of their offspring, are truisms
taught by every stud in the kingdom.   All that exists
among us, descended from the great forefather of the Turf,
are capable of producing offspring of equal pretension, as
regards the root from which they are sprung.   Far different was the result in relation to the importations of
Eastern blood contemporary with the Godolphin, and the
same it has been with all more recently introduced.
Enough, at all events, has been adduced, if not to *prove*
my position, to warrant me, at least, in its assumption, as
well as for offering it to the consideration of those who

* Annals of the British Turf, from the Introduction of Eastern blood
to the present Time.   The first century concluded in the Old Sporting
Magazine.

hold the subject to which it relates of sufficient interest to engage their attention.

From such speculations on the origin of the British race-horse, we will turn to the annals of his exploits,—a theme more generally attractive, though intrinsically less important. Here, to begin with the early worthies of the turf, all is as obscure as is the genealogical problem with which we have been already engaged. Of the performances of Childers, detailed, as they are, with all apparent microscopic observations of the seconds' hand, I am convinced that we know rather worse than nothing. In a recent work of more than an ordinary character on the subject to which it addresses itself (Lawrence's History of the Horse), Childers—Flying Childers, as he was designated *par excellence*—is stated to have been a chestnut, whereas he was a rich bay with four white legs. The same slovenly style, no doubt, attaches to the records of the early performances, as well as to the more recent attempts of equestrian historians. Again, the only criterion by which we can estimate them is, when we can refer to a timed race, because, knowing little of the principals, we cannot be supposed to have a better knowledge of the pretensions of their contemporaries. Now, even in our day, when all the appliances for chronometrical accuracy are so vastly improved and multiplied, we rarely hear of the time of a race being kept at all, even accidentally: it is never done by authority, or on a principle deserving of confidence.

We know that the taste, in the middle of the last century, inclined to long distances, and repeated exertion— six and eight-mile heats being events of constant recurrence; and yet we are required to believe that there existed at and previous to that time a flight of speed unknown to our degenerate days. Moreover, by far the greater portion of the early racers were under-sized, Galloways as the old Calendars have them in every page; and stride is, save in rare exceptions, indispensable to a high degree of swiftness. In the absence of any actual data as to speed, worthy being confided in, it may not be inconvenient to relate a performance of one of the first-class horses of that period; and, by contrasting it with a match against time, done by a contemporary hackney, some deduction may be drawn of the qualities of the racers of that era.

Gimcrack, a gray horse bred in 1760, by Cripple out of Miss Elliot, was considered one of the best of his day. In consequence of his superiority, he was sent to France, where he was matched for a large sum to do a certain distance against time. Whatever it was, he was the winner, having accomplished twenty-three miles in fifty-five minutes. This was probably in 1770. In 1778, a foundered hackney, aged twenty-two, belonging to a Mr. Hanks, did twenty-two miles within the hour, upon the high road in the neighborhood of London. Gimcrack carried eight stone: the weight on the hackney is not given, but there is no reason for believing it less than eight stone; so that one of the best race-horses of that day could only beat a broken-down hack a mile and five minutes in an hour!

It is a conventional fallacy to attribute to past days virtues superior to those in which we live. Every thing, from the seasons to the flavor of home-brewed, was better, if we credit the popular voice, "in the good old times." To examine the application of this rule to the matter before us, I may perhaps be permitted to borrow a leaf out of my own book, seeing that I could scarce make my argument stronger in any other form of words.

"After a careful examination of all the best authorities bearing upon the condition of the Turf in that so emphatically called its palmiest era—the middle of the last century—I find nothing to warrant the belief that, as a species, the contemporaries of King Herod, Imperator, Eclipse, Florizel, and Highflyer, possessed either speed, power, or symmetry, unknown to the racer of our day. At the very date to which this extraordinary excellence is ascribed, we find the degeneracy of that particular breed the subject of legislative consideration; and in 1740 that an Act of Parliament was passed, denouncing the Turf as the cause of the growing debasement of the breed of horses all over the kingdom, and fixing the weights to be carried in all plates and matches at ten stone for five-year-olds, eleven stone for six, and twelve stone for seven-year-olds and upwards, on pain of a penalty of £200, and forfeiture of the horse. It is true that this Act was repealed soon afterwards, through the intervention, as it was believed, of the Duke of Cumberland; nevertheless it is manifest that there must have existed strong grounds for complaint against the system of breeding and racing before the consideration of its economy would be made a subject of Parliamentary interference. Let us turn to the weights carried by two-year-olds fifty years ago, and those common to the present period—the former averaging from six stone to six stone six pounds, the latter from eight stone five pounds to eight stone seven pounds, and what evidence of degeneracy does that furnish?" Racing, wherever we meet it existing as a popular sport, is the growth of a root indigenous to England. All the appliances of civilization are carried to a higher degree of perfection among us, in the present day, than at any former period of our history : the Turf, and all its *materiel*, it cannot be doubted, has attained a comparative condition of excellence.

In a nation peculiarly attached to rural sports, that, as
24*

matter of course, becomes entitled to the place of honor which diffuses the greatest portion of enjoyment to the greatest number of people. In this view, racing is well entitled to the pre-eminence which it has so long claimed, and had conceded to it; but it prefers demands of a higher nature than its mere pleasurable results. In a political sense, it is an engine of no mean importance. A state must benefit largely from an agency which exhibits its nobles promoting, at great individual cost, a sport in which all classes can participate equally with themselves, and which brings together all the divisions of society for one end and purpose—social recreation. Where shall we seek the great moral of England's power and station?—In the wealth which commerce pours upon her shores?—In her wooden walls?—In the skill, learning, and valor of her sons? We can scarce study it in a more impressive page than that yearly spread before us at the great popular re-unions of Epsom, Ascot, and Doncaster. Let such as love such lore, then, search after it where the examination will surely reward their industry: we will take it up, abstract-edly, as a pastime, and in that character look into the na-ture and influence of its present economy.

As a treasury of art, an assembly or learning, ingenuity, and pleasure, our metropolis has many rivals—some su-periors: in our rural life we stand alone. Mainly this has been brought about by—is the consequence of—a general taste for field sports. Whether the cause of morality is served by horse-racing, it is not our province to inquire. An inelegant but most *apropos* salt-water axiom says, "every man to his post, and the cook to the fore-sheet." Mankind, since the creation, has set its face against all work and no play, and will do so to the end of the chapter. We are of the disciples or Democritus; and, feeling in the vein, will just touch in here, merely in outline, a faint sketch of a DERBY DAY.

Perhaps, with one exception alone, none of the realities of life come up to the anticipations of them; and what, you ask, is that singular deviation from the general rule?—It is a DERBY DAY. Imagine a conglomeration of two millions of souls stirred to its *penetralia*, shaken from its propriety, morally earthquaked, because of the necessity which annually requires that a certain portion of the mass (say a fortieth) should rendezvous in a neighborhood where certain horses are to contend some two minutes and sundry seconds for certain moneys, and you arrive at a general idea of something by no means in the ordinary course. The scene of this commotion is London, the majority of actors automata that make yearly one solitary diversion (in both the word's interpretations) from the regular cycles of their orbits. But such a Saturnalia demands a word anent its note of preparation.

As soon as the month dawns, big with the catastrophe of Epsom Races, straightway from Belgrave Square to Shoreditch, from the Regent's Park to uttermost Rotherhithe, forth the sackage goes that guts, from garret to cellar, every Pantechnicon, Bazaar, and Repository of all and singular the wheeled conveniences and inconveniences peculiar to each. Anon the horse, in all its infinite gradations, is had in requisition, from Newman's choicest specimens of blood, that devour the Surry highways, to the living quadrupedal skeleton redeemed from the knacker's knife at the last Smithfield show for fifteen shillings, and a "drop o' summit for luck." The day arrives, and lo! a mighty chain of carriages, "in linked grumbling long drawn out," extends from the Elephant and Castle to the merry Downs of Epsom, witherwards we will suppose thy anxious way hath at length been achieved. The moisture of travel encumbereth thy brow: searchest thou for thy best Bandana to relieve thee of the damp? Luckless wight!—

> "——— That handkerchief
> Did an Egyptian from thy pocket prig."

Is not the tide of humanity at the flood of spring? Ten deep do vehicles of all kinds, definite and undefinable, line the course. Opposite and around the stand all is high-bred and aristocratic: lower down, leading for Tattenham's classic corner, you haply take your curious path. What lots of pretty girls you encounter as you go! —each so lady-like and *bien mise*, you would never dream of their metropolitan whereabouts, were it not for those awful mortalities that cluster around them; brothers, cousins, lovers it may be—pale shadows that haunt the glimpses of Bow Church—horrible illusions from Ludgate Hill and the Ward of Cheap, with prickly frills to their linen, swallow tails to their coats, green velvet waistcoats, or, still more shocking, similar habiliments of black satin, whereon the indecent chain of Mosaic grins ghastly, like the gilding on a coffin!—faugh!

Drawing near to the lines, hark! from glass coach, britscha, jarvey, phaeton, proceed various sounds of discontent.—" Cold chickens, veal pie, lobsters and *no* salt." —" Half-a-dozen bottles is all very fine, and never no corkscrew."—" Sir, I'll set that right if you'll only accommodate us with the loan of a glass; really it's too provoking."
. . . . . Ascend the hill, approach the Ring, and hear what sums are jeopardied on the coming event!—enough to purchase half-a-score of German principalities! but the warren is open, and thither you are borne by the countless

thousands who throng for a glance of the coursers on whom
hang the hopes and fears of all.

No spot can be better adapted for the purpose to which
it is assigned than the so well-known warren; but all that
nature has done man takes especial care to frustrate. Instead of its cool quiet alleys being kept for the tranquil
preparation of animals peculiarly disposed to excitement,
(their most dangerous foe at a moment when the entire
possession of every faculty is of such vital consequence,)
every "dingle, nook, and bosky bourn" is invaded by a
horde of ravenous, sight-seeing cockneys, of all beasts of
prey the most reckless and perverse. Amid this restless
crowd of babbling, cigar-smoking untameables, the process
of saddling is effected, and, with graceful steps, the fiery-
footed adversaries depart for the lists.

You reach the place of starting, and what awaits you
there? Order, decorum, and all fitting arrangement for
the important essay of which it is the arena? A second
chaos!—all the human elements thrown together in a moral
whirlpool. A score of men in buckram suits, (blue linsey-
woolsey,) attempting to dispose of twice as many thousands
—something like barring the gates of a beleagued town
with boiled carrots! They draw together for the start—
infinitely the most influential point in the great game to be
played. Here all is confusion worse confounded: the mul-
titude opens its thousand throats of brass; the steeds are
frantic; the jockeys (born and bred devils from their
cradle) practise every conceivable stratagem ever hatched
in Fiendom; and there stands one nervous old man to front
the pitiless pelting, and produce from such materials a result with which all are to be satisfied. "They are off!"
and the old gentleman, in his agony, pronounces "Go,"
and the fatal signal has gone forth. Over the hill, adown

the fall, there is a meteoric flash, as though a rainbow had borrowed the wings of the lightning, and all is over!

The Derby is decided—the steeds turned round—the jockeys approach the scales—Holy Mother of Moses! has it entered the heart of man (even an Irishman) to conceive the tearing and swearing, the howling and screeching, that instant rends the empyrean! Quick as thought a circle of bludgeons and constables is formed, into which the horses as they arrive are received, and against which a roaring ocean of humanity is dashing as fiercely as the vexed Atlantic. Look towards the grand stand—behold whole acres of countenances uplifted to the sky, wedged as closely as a crate of French eggs, and resembling nothing as yet discovered but a monstrous dish of opened oysters! The round earth is shaken, and echo gives up the ghost—the thunder hides its diminished head, as with the bellowings of ten thousand volcanoes, myriads of furious lungs crash forth, "WHO HAS WON?" Thus whilom did I sing of this scene; and with better experience, save in the episodes of flying voltigeurs, men "with never no back-bones at all, only a slip of gristle to hold head and heels together," and epicures in cutlery, "who swallow knives and forks for all the world like gingerbread nuts," I can add nothing to the *beau ideal* of a DERBY DAY.

How little can they, who first give existence to a principle, foresee how it will operate, and what may be its results. The pastime of horse-racing, fostered and promoted simply as a channel of amusement by the gay and thoughtless Charles, called into being the strongest impulse of man's nature—emulation, and thus entailed upon this country a race of the noblest of all existing animals, of a character apparently superior to that originally destined by nature. This may be an erroneous theory, but as yet we are unacquainted with any variety of the horse comparable to the artificial stock known as our thorough-blood. The very general efforts that were made from that period by the nobles and great landed proprietors to improve by lavish outlay, and all the appliances which it can command, the best strains of the recently imported Oriental blood, towards the middle of the last century, seem to have carried the race-horse, *as a species*, as near to perfection as his generic organization will admit. True, every year produced some few infinitely superior to their contemporaries, but they were phenomena,—indebted to no individuality of parentage for their excellence, and unpossessed of the faculty of endowing their descendants with similar gifts. As a race, when opposed to the indigenous horse of any quarter of the earth, the English thorough-blood is universally victorious; among the various families into which it is divided at home, no *constant* succession of superiority has ever discovered itself.

I am aware that those who only take a superficial view of the economy of our racing system, will at once pronounce against this position. They will adduce the sons and daughters of King Herod, Eclipse, and Highflyer; in our day, of Sultan and Emilius, as far surpassing the ordinary run of their contemporaries. But they do not bear in mind that not only did and does the progeny of these justly celebrated sires greatly outnumber that of their less favored brothers, but that the best mares of their respective eras were and are exclusively put to them. Not to travel beyond our own day for proofs, did excellence ensure its like, what chance would have remained to those who now and then breed a solitary nomination against the gigantic studs of Hampton Court, Riddlesworth, or Underly? To confine the question to the present year, (1838,) we had evidence that not all the wealth, skillful training, Sybarite care and treatment of the best of England's blood could produce a match for the son of one of our indifferent racers, —the despised of an Irish tenth-rate stable,—the wonderful and the basely-abused Harkaway.* I may be told that he was defeated here, and by second-raters, too,—but under what circumstances? With ordinary care, without having been subjected to actual ill-treatment, at weight for age there was nothing of the year in England that could have stood any chance with him.

From these premises the deduction at which we arrive bearing upon the economy of the turf, its nature and influence is twofold, and admits of a very brief solution,—the first being that the day is long passed since the means of winning upon the race-course were to be obtained by breeding; the second, that the vast advantages still to be derived from a proper application of our thorough-blood is most strangely neglected. Mr. Bowes began his racing career by breeding a winner of the Derby, while the late Duke of Leeds, the most extensive breeder of blood stock in the north, toiled in vain for the Leger till he won it with a colt bought from the tail of the plough. Lord George Bentinck, the best winner on the turf of modern days, if the Calendar be any criterion, regards breeding racers as an expedient no man in his senses should dream of, and, acting upon his theory, has put money in his purse. A first-class racer, a colt of extraordinary promise, are each productions of chance-medley, only to be come at by being secured where and when they can be found.

But if the Turf be thus restricted in further profiting,

* This extraordinary animal is now (December, 1838,) advertised for sale, his price six thousand guineas, with this strange addition, "that his owner (Mr. Ferguson) rides him hunting once or twice a week!"

save as matter of hazard, by the means which securely ministered to the success of its first speculators, it furnishes materials from which may be moulded other distinct races, as valuable, each in its province, as the flying family of the modern race-course, now the sole representatives of our thorough-blood. The ragged regiment of cock-tails will, it is devoutly to be hoped, speedily be disbanded; the day soon arrive when no gentleman shall be seen bestriding the mongrel of a base-bred hackney, scarce worthy the shafts of a costermonger's trap. And first, as is befitting, such reform must commence with its next of kin—THE FIELD. Shall this, assuredly the second—nay, the twin-sport of racing, in the esteem of Englishmen, long continue dependent upon chance for a supply of horses for its service? Impossible; the period cannot be far distant in which the British thorough-bred hunter will be as distinct a race, and of as high renown, as his progenitors were the pride of the Turf.

25

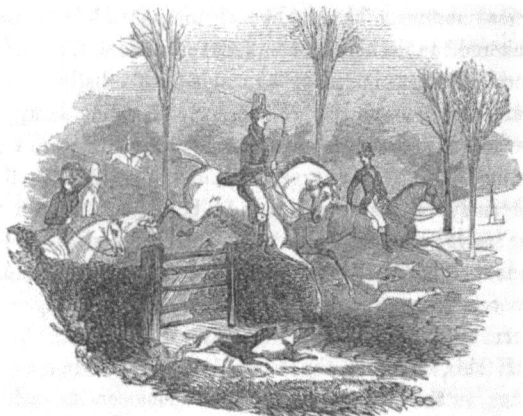

HUNTING.

As the whole object of the Manly Exercises is not accomplished in the attainment and practice of them, it was thought convenient that the business of their details should be succeeded by a partial notice of some of those sports of which they form the elementary process, and which may be regarded as their ultimate " end and aim." It has been well said by my talented friend, Nimrod, that all the writing in the world will not make a sportsman. The pen of Pindar, and the pencil of Grant, indeed, exhibit him in all perfection to our admiration; but, could they both write for the education of the student whose ambition is Olympic fame, they would not insure success. Like the poet, he must be born, in a manner, to his cunning.

The Exercises, upon which Mr. Walker has written, admitted of being inculcated by methodical rules, and acquired by a systematic routine of practice. An acquaintance with them will be found of service to youth, whatever the desti-

nation of its manhood may be; while they are essential to
the formation of a frame and character fitted for the maturity likely to be devoted to the wear and tear of our hardy
Rural Sports. Driving and Yachting, though neither of
them strictly coming within the pale of a course of physical exercises, still are not out of place in a practical book
devoted to the science of manly recreations, because each
is governed by certain rules, which may be taught and acquired. It is not so with the subjects constituting the
matter on which we are at present engaged. A man may
out-study Zoroaster without being one whit the better
qualified for winning a fifty pound plate, hitting off the line
of a fox that has been headed, or bringing down his wood-
cock in cover; these are arts which, being decimated, leave
one part to theory and nine in favor of practice. For this
cause I have made my Article on the Turf of a character
more suited to the purposes of the general reader than those
of the visionary theorist, who may fondly hope to meet, on
page traced by mortal hands, a recipe for breeding, training, and managing an embryo winner of Derby or Leger.
The Chase, however, admits of a certain code of general
maxims: it has, if not limits, at all events courses better
defined than those of the Turf, and to the application of
them by practical men of modern experience we will at once
proceed.

Assuming that a tolerable proficiency in horsemanship
has been attained before the young disciple of Diana ven-
tures to show at all with hounds, he will do well to dedi-
cate the first of his novitiate to hare-hunting, whether his
future destination be that of a M. F. H., or merely a parta-
ker of the "light from heaven," dispensed by the "noble
science." As this little treatise addresses itself more particularly to the latter, it will be sufficient to point out what

should be his aim in his early lessons. Of these, the most
essential to the formation of a good sportsman, and the only
one that will enable any man to live to the end of a severe
run, is, that he cultivate the faculty of a *quick eye to
hounds.* With harriers he will constantly have practice in
this task : the perpetual doubles to which nine hares out of
ten, when chased, resort, will soon convince him of the necessity of keeping a wary look out for the line towards
which the leading hounds incline. He will have little difficulty in deciding with which portion of the pack, or with
which individual of it, the scent is, if he only observe
closely when there is any indication of a check. The
instant a hound catches the scent, he will see him drop his
tail horizontally, and spring to the front, the one who has
lost it elevating his, as if engaged in questing. Keeping
his look-out always upon the leaders, and leaving the body
of the pack to follow a similar system, he turns his horse
as he sees the chase lean, and thus is going at his ease *inside* the circle, around which others can hardly live at the
best their nags can accomplish. When a huntsman is
coming past with hounds,—particularly at check in a lane
or road,—get out of his way all you can ; the narrower the
pass the greater the necessity that you give room, or hounds
must break over the fence, and so run the risk of putting
up, or crossing the line of, another hare : moreover, horses
on such occasions are apt to strike out at hounds, and it is
far from pleasant to be constituted by such a casualty "the
observed of all observers."

In the matter of riding at fences, with harriers you will
be more enabled to suit your practice to the individual case
than when you come to ride alongside fox-hounds. With
the former, when any thing very cramp crosses your line,
you may "look before you leap," and this is no bad maxim,

whoever may choose to sneer at it. Let this too be an
axiom from which you never depart, as far as regards the
hounds: when you are out with the jolly dogs, "hear and
see, and say nothing"—so shall you earn golden opinions
from the field in general, and prevent much out-pouring of
wrath from the officials in particular. It will serve you to
bear in mind that in almost every difficulty of ground a
horse can serve himself better than you can assist him. I
do not mean to say that in heavy, deep galloping you should
not hold him together, and if there be a furrow or path at
hand, that you should not give him the advantage of it.
But in woodland, for instance, where young timber has been
felled, and the surface is covered with live stubs, give him
his head: let him pick his own way; never touch his
mouth with the bridle to guide him, and you will find how
rarely he will give a chance away. Thus in a rabbit warren the difficulty is doubled by the nervous man who
attempts to steer his horse. The biped is looking at one
hole, the quadruped at another, and being diverted from the
spot where he intended to place his foot, puts it *in* where it
was meant that he should not. Still, however, you may
attempt it: never charge ground of this nature without
using the precaution of slacking your pace. I remember a
well-known bruising rider, who thought it impossible that
he could be hurt, once trying the experiment over a warren
in the neighborhood of Whitchurch, in Shropshire, and
being assured of the affirmative in the first hundred yards
by the fracture of his collar-bone, and the dislocation of a
shoulder.

With the common run of fences, where the grip is from
you, go faster at them than when it lies on the side you
take off from. When they consist of live thorns and quicks
newly laid down, take them, whenever the chance presents

25*

itself, *aslant*, rising where the top of the thorn is laid, as
being the least capable of holding your horse's knees,
should they catch in rising at it. In your novitiate it is
hardly necessary to offer you any advice as to water. As
a general rule, however, it may as well be said here as elsewhere that, in brook-jumping, pace comes first and then
judgment. With a powerful impetus you get over; should
your horse blunder, somehow—if with a fall at the other
side, no matter: less speed enables you to pick your ground
better, but it throws all the odds on the side of a cold-bath,
should the span be wider than you calculated on, or the
bank be soft, and let you in. Never take hold of your
horse's head till you feel that he is safely landed; if there
is a scramble for it, and you pull at him but an ounce, it
may turn the beam of his equipoise, and in you go together.

Young hands are prone to think that it is necessary to
the acquisition of the reputation of a sportsman that they
show in front throughout a run. Indeed, I might have
said this idea seems to hold with many who ought to be
wiser. The sooner the youthful Nimrod discards this
fallacy the better. The chances are so multiplied and
various against a good run that it is next to a miracle how
a real clipper ever occurs. From foil, to which ground is
everywhere exposed, down to an infant of three years old
that heads your quarry, on every side you are beset with
risk, even *with* a scent. Without it your difficulty becomes
almost an impossibility, and that is the time when over-
riding, more fatal than all other obstacles put together, is
to be seen in its superlative degree. There is your hard-
rider, *par excellence*, who *will* be first; the leader pulls up
at a check—the nuisance passes him, even with hounds at
fault, without a moment's care for the mischief he must do
the chase, or what he may do himself. Let such as this

teach you that which you should avoid : acquire in youth
the way you should go, and in your maturity you will not
depart from it.

We now come to the matriculation of the " noble science,"
and consider the *quondam* novice entered to fox-hunting.
It would be bootless here to offer any eulogy upon a sport
admitted, by authorities allowing no question, to be, in a
political as well as a social view, a powerful moral engine.
In a letter now before me, which I lately received from a
gallant general, himself a master of fox-hounds, he ascribes
to a taste for the chase that characteristic manly daring
which distinguishes the officers of our service from those
of any other. Of all field sports, its claims are the most
general upon the properties of manhood. The tiger-hunts
of the East may appeal more directly to the courage, but
with activity and physical endurance they have little or
nothing to do. But see the qualities that must combine
to form the accomplished fox hunter. He must be bold,
ready, decisive, capable of commanding and sustaining
great bodily exertion : he must join unity of purpose to
promptness of action ; capability of foreseeing events, that
he may best turn them to advantage, with a frame and a
spirit alike competent to meet and oppose undauntedly
difficulties and dangers, how and when they may assail
him. I would not have it supposed that I claim for the
chase a higher station for enterprise than any other of the
adventurous occupations in which we find mankind employed. It would be absurd for an instant, for example,
to compare it with that most exciting and magnificent of
all the daring offices to which man has ever addressed
himself—the South Sea fishing. But as a sport,—an act
to which pleasure alone induces him, fox-hunting has
nothing at all bearing comparison with it in modern days.

To the present fashion of its details we will now turn our consideration.

I do not think it necessary here to enter into any foreign matter, such as the nature and economy of the establishment with which the field may be taken with reference to the country hunted, or the number of days weekly to be devoted to its business. We will suppose our young Nimrod has completed all such arrangements in a convenient fashion, and proceed to the *res gesta* for which he has made preparation. In this hard riding era, it is regarded as a dashing style of going to cover, by your aspiring tyro, to approach it as the crow would fly. If he *must* go thither across country, let him, at all events, avoid passing through or riding too near any of the covers likely to be drawn during the day. If they hold a good fox, it is sure notice for him to quit, for he is ever on the *qui vive*. The result is, should the hounds be thrown in, they come upon a scent some hours old—crawl upon it over probably the cream of the country, never come on terms with him; and a capital day's sport is lost to a whole field by a selfish half hour's lark. Arrived at the place of meeting, he should not address himself to the master, if he hunt his own hounds; or, in the other case, to the huntsman, notwithstanding he may be on familiar terms with them, beyond the mere exchange of a passing civility. Even then, a man, bent upon showing a good day's sport, has his mind sufficiently engaged on the business before him. He is consulting temporary causes, by which to be directed as to the particular cover to begin with, and how it is to be drawn. The point of wind, the nature of the day, the weather of the preceding week,—all must be weighed, and brought to assist his judgment. A fox well found is always the most likely to be well accounted for.

But if conversation with the master or huntsman be inconvenient before hounds are thrown off, afterwards it becomes a positive impertinence. It is no excuse for doing so that they are not actually engaged at the moment. A huntsman, having drawn without a find, is probably waiting for some of his hounds; at the same time he is debating with himself what cover he shall next try, and how to get to it, as the wind may affect the best lying in it for his fox. He has also observed how his hounds have behaved, and has orders to give to a whip as to the conduct of some one prone to riot; or that a particular corner of the cover about being drawn shall be carefully watched. In short, success or failure are dependent on his management: and how can he deliberate if he is to stand a general catechism?

If it be a large cover, keep within hearing of the hounds and huntsman. This can only be effected by being down wind, and should be done without any reference to the distance round, which it may impose. Of course, it is not intended that a man should take anything he can avoid out of his horse by galloping round a cover, but let him keep on steadily opposite the hounds, taking heed that he does not get so far forward as to endanger heading back the fox, and so spoiling his own and his neighbours' sport. This I only recommend where covers are very large, and even then it may not be the best system. In all cases where it is practicable, I never throw a chance away by losing sight of hounds. I remember, some years ago, meeting Sir Richard Puleston at Cresford village, whence we trotted to a wood that skirts the high road to Chester. As we jogged forward, a friend overtook me, accosting me with, "You need not hurry yourself, for they'll find nothing where they're going: it has been beaten within an hour by a party of coursers, who have left nothing alive on four

legs within it, you may rely." In ten minutes, the pack
and field were streaming, best pace, after a fox found in
that same coppice, away for Shavington, over a country
like the cream of Leicestershire or Northampton.

In fox-hunting, depend solely upon yourself, and keep
with the pack. Even in going from cover to cover, be
with them. Circumstances frequently arise, which induce
a huntsman to abandon trying a place upon which he may
have previously fixed; and how often has a fox jumped
out of a hedgerow in the centre of a pack trotting indus-
triously away to look for a chance probably half a dozen
miles off! In windy weather, when hounds are in cover,
unless you draw it with them, it is two to one you never
get away at all, and ten to one against a good start. I
have had some experience of horses in my day, and have
ever found, that, of all ways of beating them, the surest is
that of trying to catch hounds. Laying aside the excitement and energy produced by the music, alongside of which
they go sailing away in wild delight, it must be remembered that the pace of fox hounds with a scent is equal to
the best, if not superior, that any first class hunter possesses. What sort of a nag then is it, that you can expect
to catch them with ten minutes' law? In calm weather,
also, the danger of losing sight of hounds is by no means
to be disregarded. There are some days (those which
invariably carry the best scent) when hounds will find, and
fly away like magic, not one in the pack attempting to
throw tongue. Here, if the cover be large, unless you
have them in your eye, the odds are you never get away;
and see what you loose—the excellence of the scent has
stopped the cry: the faster hounds go, the less they say
about it.

When in a large cover, with hounds unavoidably out of

sight, depend upon your ear much rather than upon the movements of others. You will constantly find men riding straight on end, merely because the hounds were running so when they entered, while very probably the fox has turned short, and is already away, with the pack at his brush, in an opposite direction. With a little patience and attention, your ear will soon come to the knack of detecting the line of hounds in cover: it is well worth your while to take pains to acquire this art. When you *have* learnt it, you will speedily find out the advantage it will confer upon your horse, and yourself too. It is by no means easy to lay down rules for that which so mainly depends upon circumstances; but it may be convenient to offer a few examples, upon which you may found a system for general application. Suppose, for instance, you have had a burst with your fox, and he has reached a large cover, in which there are strong earths, or beyond which lies a country too open for a blown fox to set his head for. If the earths are open, in he goes, and there is an end of him; if stopped, he turns, or leans to the right or left. During this time, brief as it may be, you have eased your horse; he gets his wind (a minute, in many cases, will put him right after a very quick thing), and you are fresh, while your hard rider has been going best pace beyond the hounds, and comes toiling after you in vain. These points of practice, however, require good judgment, and great promptness of action. You must know well how to distinguish between a cry that grows faint and fainter, as a failing scent leads to a final check, and one that, from a crash, at once becomes almost wholly lost, as the pack flies to their fox with a view, or a scent breast high.

You will, no doubt, at the commencement of your career, hear a great deal about the influence the wind has upon the line of chase. Do not take all such theory for gospel. I have tried my hand at a few systems of the kind, but only found one that admitted general adoption. When a fox, on being found, takes up wind at first, do not ride, though the pace be first-rate, so as to take much out of your horse. Foxes constantly, after going a mile or so up wind, turn and head back. This will let you in with a good start, and a fresh nag; and even should the chase hold on up wind, you run little risk of being thrown out, as you will have the cry to guide you, and the puff in, to enable you to get to them when the first brush is over.

One good effect of the hard riding of modern days is, that hounds are much less meddled with by strangers than they used to be when first I remember fox-hunting. Indeed, I am not sure that too much etiquette does not now exist upon that point. The total disappearance of the thong to the hunting-whip seems like carrying a good thing rather too far. A fox breaks probably under your horse's nose: out comes the pack, none of the servants are at hand, and they run a field or two from the cover before any one stops them, or their own mettle allows them to turn : one crack of your whip would have saved all that. One thing you *can* do without your thong, but you should be very careful how you do it. I allude to hallooing a fox away. Never attempt to lift your voice till he is evidently bent on going, and then give him at least a field's law, or the odds are, back he goes, perhaps into the hounds' mouths. When he *is* gone, then clap your hand behind your ear, and give the " Tally-ho—*away !*" to the best of the lungs that are in you. Should he merely show for a moment outside, and then pop in again, give a "Tally-ho—back !" that it may be known where he was seen, as well as that he is not away. Another service in this latter halloo is, that all the points where it is likely he will try to break will be left clear for him. If a fox is seen crossing a ride or path, in cover, in front of you, pull up; and if hounds are at check, tally him, as it will serve as a guide to the huntsman.

In drawing a cover you may give this signal, should any fox cross you, but if you have run him in, be awake not to tally any but the hunted one, or you will have few thanks for your trouble. A little experience will easily teach you the difference between one just unkenneled and that which has stood any time before hounds. Not only will the former be sleek and unstained, but the method of going be very dissimilar. A fresh fox bounds off, throwing his hind legs clear from him, and his whole frame, from the tip of his nose to that of his brush, as straight as an arrow; if hunted, and at all blown or beaten, his action is labored, like that of a rocking-horse, his back is curved, his brush drooping, and the ears thrown back, all the fire for which when found, his eye is so remarkable, quenched, and exchanged for an air of cunning and subdued resolution. I am far from any design of counselling you to interfere with the business of a pack of fox-hounds that you may be either in the habit of hunting with, or one that you may merely meet by accident occasionally. Still there are instances in which to withhold all assistance would be to put the chance of sport in jeopardy, and in which the true lover of the chase ought to act first and think afterwards. Should any casualty, for example, so find you that, *with hounds at fault,* you catch a halloo that the huntsman does not or cannot hear, contrive so to place yourself between the halloo and the hounds that you may be heard by huntsman or pack, and so lead them on the line that the halloo proceeds from. I repeat, however,

26

that these and similar aids must be offered with due discretion. The halloo may be a false one—true, but had
you gone to make inquiries, you, too, would have been out
of hearing—the points of fox-hunting require temporary
and local adaptation, and a head-piece to direct all. Mere
physical endowments will never make an accomplished
fox-hunter—combined with judgment they are very excellent subsidiaries : for him who would shine in the chase

"Orandum est, ut sit mens sana in corpore sano."

In riding to hounds it will essentially serve you if you
bear in mind what ninety-nine out of a hundred seem never
to give a thought to, namely, that the pack only acts *pro tanto*
upon the line of country which a fox is likely to take. Independent of the point which it is assumed he will make
for, he has a hundred other things to avoid, as well as the
enemies baying on his trail. He settles his point, but he
must also get to it unseen. Unless beaten and all but run
into, he will give a wide berth to any thing like the habi-
tation of man as well as man himself. Thus, by keeping
your eye well before you, there is a chance that the turn
hounds will take, may be so far anticipated, that you avoid
riding outside of their circle. It has been well said that
when hounds are running, a man ought to consider what,
under the circumstances in which things happen to be, he
would do were he the fox. I cannot offer you better
counsel. By adopting such a principle you will be enabled
to foresee a check should you detect any thing in the line
that the chase is taking, however far ahead—and if you
have a knowledge of the country, you will calculate such
chances almost to a certainty. In a district with which you
are acquainted, the line a fox takes when found, will enable
you to judge whether he has been before hunted, and if

he has, the odds are he runs the same again. Even in cover you may fairly assume that he is accustomed to be stirred by the ring he takes, the points he tries, the gaps he uses in the fences, and similar observations, which should be the business on which you are intent from the moment the hounds are thrown in.

More than once it has been my good fortune to secure a clipping run for a sporting field by keeping a clear look-out upon the matter at issue, *and nothing else*, when a long series of covers drawn blank, and such dampers, have sent one-half of the morning's muster home, while the other had taken *to the dernier resort* of cigars and gossip. As an instance of this, several years ago, with the Shropshire, when Mr. Cresset Pelham had them, we had been at it from the hour of meeting till past three, in November too, and no luck. Having trotted on to our last hope for the day, it was tried, and pronounced—blank ! Already twilight had commenced, the huntsman outside the cover was blowing his horn, the pack mustered, and home was the order of march. I had watched the gathering with care ; and, as we were already trotting from the side of the spinny, it struck me that an old and favorite bitch was missing. I called the huntsman's attention to it. There was a pause— a faint wimple was heard in the still valley—anon it opened into a cry, " Hark to it !"—the pack flew to the challenge —there was a mighty crash : in a minute a fox broke away in sight of every man who had had the patience to await the last throw on the dice. A burst of twenty minutes was the result, without a pull from best pace ; and we turned him up in the open just as the parish lantern gave us notice to look out for squalls.

There exists, in some masters of hounds, a disposition to keep back such men as, when hounds are in chase, follow

through the covers they take in their line. It is not my
desire to inculcate disobedience to the powers that be; but
certainly I cannot second that principle, either with reference to those who adopt it, or those to whom it is intended
to apply. When a hunted fox has reached a cover, not
only is it the best way to cheer hounds to him, that they
should not feel themselves alone, but also the noise made
by men following them is the most likely way to make a
fresh fox break, without any of the stragglers getting on
him. I have seen a fox crawl into cover dead beat, and
already in the mouths of the pack. The huntsman and a
whip followed them—the "whoo-whoop" was given—the
master and the rest of the field waited on the outside.
They remained in patience till ten minutes had elapsed.
"Surely," said an old hand at last, "they are doing more
than baying him with all that cry. Hark! it has got to
the opposite side of the wood:—by heavens! they're away
with a fresh fox." And so they were; and they killed him
at the end of forty minutes without a check, and without a
sight of them ever being caught, save by the servants, who
had followed to lift the fox that had crawled dead beat into
the cover.

I have thus attempted to sketch, for the young disciple
of the "noble science," a slight code of maxims of general
application. For the principles of practice to direct him
in the constantly occurring cases, which admit of no rule
save that arising out of individual circumstances, he must
rely upon himself. Under this general head of HUNTING,
I have not thought it necessary to enter upon any varieties
of the chase, save those of the fox and the hare. Stag-
hunting, as a rural sport, is limited to a very few districts;
and for its pursuit requires only a knowledge of horsemanship, and a quick eye to a country. Fox-hunting and hare-

hunting I have treated with reference only to the points of practice which apply to the convenience of those who select them as appliances of recreation. This work, in its nature, is rudimentary: it professes to deal with the elements of our manly exercises, and so far to treat of our national sports of RACING, HUNTING, and SHOOTING. Its office is to instruct the beginner, leaving the higher classes to volumes of more pretension. With this view of its purpose, I have brought the subject of the Chase to the limit which I designed for it. It is a truly manly—a noble sport. Long may it be cherished and fostered in our land! The qualities which it calls into action are those which confer honor on manhood,—courage, promptness, activity, and decision. Surely these are rare properties in which to exercise a youth, and these the Chase will engender and nourish: while to such as require that a moral attach to every occupation of life, it has this to recommend it, that, in riding to hounds, this great truth is hourly inculcated —"Honesty is the best policy."

26*

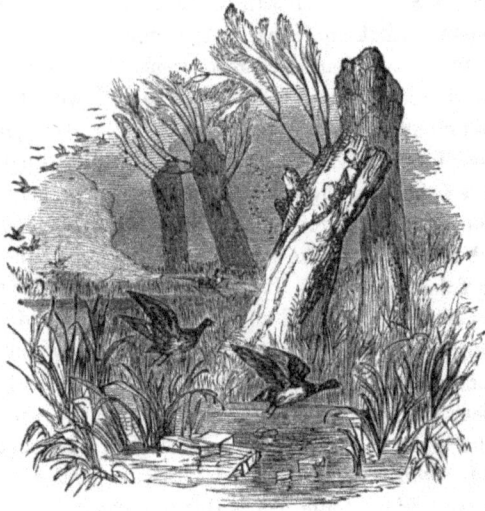

SHOOTING.

It is my purpose, in the present chapter, as in the two preceding, to offer, as companion to the system of exercises described in the first part of this work, certain practical rules upon another of those popular field sports, a knowledge of which has in all ages been considered, in this country, part of a gentleman's education. The perfection to which we have attained in the manufacture of all the implements connected with this branch of sporting, would make a dissertation on the *materiel* of shooting a piece of useless information to those for whose service these notices are intended. Instead, therefore, of filling these pages with elaborate instructions for selecting his guns, gun-cases, flasks, belts, and the whole catalogue of shooting gear, I present my reader with one solitary golden maxim, which will in-

sure to him the possession of a perfect apparatus, and that
eventually on the most economical terms : Let him go, for
every article of his equipment, to the most celebrated artist
in the item of which he has need. It is true that, compared with the scale of prices in the provinces, the charges
of the first-rate London gunmakers are startling things
upon paper, and so are those made by coachmakers of the
same class. Indeed, the same may be said of the rate of
demand common to the leading dealers of the metropolis ;
but he will find that *finis coronat opus*. An economical
friend of mine, who was recently quartered in Ireland, ordered, of one of the most respectable firms in Dublin, a
travelling chariot, the price, with the usual *et ceteras*, being
two hundred and fifty pounds : here it would have cost him
three hundred, or three hundred and twenty. Just as it
was completed, he was ordered home ; and his new bargain
broke down with him fourteen times between Liverpool and
London. As a contrast to this : An old sporting associate,
never particularly distinguished for his thrift, recently show-
ed me a pair of shooting shoes, for which he paid Hoby two
guineas, that he has had in constant work for sixteen years !
No record has been preserved of the number of times they
have had new bottoms. The only perishable portions of
these cordwaining phenomena, however, are their *soles:*
their bodies appear to be immortal.

To return to the appointments of the young aspirant to
the honors of the trigger. Although I set out with supposing him equipped with the best double detonator that
money can procure from a maker of known character, and
all other mechanical appliances for the field, a proper management and judicious arrangement of them is by no means
to be similarly obtained. Upon the condition of those mechanical aids his success depends, quite as much as the

adroitness to which he may arrive in the use of them. Whether that department be in the hands of a game-keeper fully competent to all its details, or there be an actual necessity for the master's eye to direct it, a knowledge of the most approved means will be found equally essential. Proficiency in any art or science requires an intimacy with the whole machinery of its economy. It was this conviction that made an emperor a laborer in a dockyard, and should induce every sportsman to acquaint himself with the minutest particulars bearing upon his craft. To this end I will give a few rules, derived as well from personal experience as from some of the most approved authorities on the subject that have appeared in print.

GUN-CLEANING.—Use cold water for the purpose of cleansing the barrel, and finish by pouring in boiling water, taking care to stop the touch-hole. Shake it up and down well, and drain it from the muzzle, which will clear the chamber. The hot water greatly aids the process of drying,—one of the most important parts of gun-washing. After the washing is concluded, by looking down the barrel with the touch-hole open, you will be enabled to see into the chamber, and ascertain whether it be effectually cleared out or otherwise. The foulness of the barrel of course must be the criterion by which the person employed in cleaning it will be decided. Should it require to be scoured, to remove powder encrusted on its sides, very fine sand and hot water should be used, and care taken to rinse it out thoroughly, at the last, with boiling water, to clear the chamber of anything that may have been driven into it by the washing-rod. The material in ordinary use for gun-cleaning is tow, to which there is the objection that particles are apt to become detached from it, and lodge in the chambers. To prevent any chance of this kind, I would recommend the substitution of cloth, which will be found to answer the purpose quite as well, being at the same time free from all such hazard. It is a bad habit to fall into, that of laying by your gun loaded: let the charge be drawn after the day's work. If you have had but a few shots, the less trouble there will be in the cleaning: a mere hot-water rinse, and a good drying, will be enough. Should your gun contain an old charge when you go out, do not put your faith in it: the odds are all in favor of its hanging fire. Squib it off, first drawing the shot, and load again while the barrels are warm; probe your touch-holes; wipe your locks within and without; and if you cannot command success afterwards, you will have the satisfaction of knowing that you have taken the best course to ensure it.

Every time you load, observe whether your touch-hole be free; it is but a moment's occupation, and a certain security against a monstrous annoyance—missing fire, probably at one of your best chances during the day. In all cases of hanging or missing fire, the seat of the disease is the touch-hole or chamber, if your cap has exploded: to these apply the remedy. I speak only with reference to detonators, as they have now become so very universal: of course when a flint gun is used, the mischief may be caused by a faulty flint. Your last act should be, when the day's sport is over, before you enter the house, to let down the springs of your locks: the less stress you keep upon them, the more power and elasticity they will retain. This is the plan to make one lock wear out the best Damascus barrel.

POWDER.—The names of most of the great manufacturers of gunpowder are now sufficient guaranty for the excellence of the article bearing their signatures. Purchase your supply from any respectable house, and you will be secure that it is genuine: beyond the label you need not seek. Your care, then, must be to preserve the original strength, by putting it into canisters closely corked and sealed, after first having carefully dried it,—a process for which Colonel Hawker gives this excellent recipe: "Your powder should always be propely *dried*, in order to do which, make *two* or *three* plates very hot before the fire, and (first taking care to wipe them well, lest any particle of cinder should adhere to them,) keep constantly shifting the powder from one to the other, without allowing it to remain sufficiently long in either to cool the plate. The powder will then be more effectually aired, and more expeditiously dried, than by the more common means of using only *one* plate, which the powder, by lying on it, soon makes cold, and therefore the plate requires to be two or three times heated." Nothing can be added to this, save the admonition that the operation · be formed at such a distance from the fire as to prevent the possibility of a spark or cinder reaching you. The surest way is to dry your powder in one room, and to heat your plates in another.

SHOT.—Here is a division of my subject much less easily disposed of than the last. The selection of shot is a question upon which many of the best authorities are at issue. Some deal with it only in reference to the game for which it is intended; others consider it merely as having relation to the length and diameter of the barrel for which it is required. I recommend the middle course,—*medio tutissimus ibis*. Colonel Hawker tells us that "it is not so much the magnitude of the pellet, as the force with which it is driven, that does the execution." No one can accord more cheerful fealty than I do to the generality of that first-rate sportman's opinions; but I cannot allow my admiration to dazzle my common sense, or to subscribe to this hypothesis. With a swan-drop you break the leg of wild-boar or red-deer; but could any force known to the science of projectiles accomplish it with a grain of number 9, or dust-shot? The rule should be, to suit your number to your game— the exception, to your gun and its calibre. Taking the average size at which fowling-pieces are now made, and the general character of English sporting, I have no hesitation in saying that there are very few instances in which number 7 will not be found to answer the purposes of a day's shooting. It is not the power to penetrate that fills the bag. Many a bird carries off a quarter of an ounce of lead in his body; but break his wing, and what can he do then? The advocate of small shot urges the increased space which it covers, and *consequently* the increased chances in favor of its hitting; but to hit your bird, and to bring him down, are two very different things. Catch him anywhere with a good-sized pellet, and the odds are that he comes to bag; stuff him with *dust*, and he flies away with a whole charge, unless it has encountered a vital part. It is to be remembered that I am not here addressing my observations to first-rate masters of the trigger,—to such professors as Ross, Sutton, or Osbaldiston. I have not deemed it necessary to go into the relative merits of shot upon such minute niceties as the increased rotatory motion of the larger pellets, and the like. In an epitomized treatise, like this, the length of my design only extends to offering the best general hints that suggest themselves to me, as applicable to the service of the novice. To such, then, I say, in all ordinary cases, make use of number 7 : never go higher, for a jack-snipe will often fly away with the full of a charger of number 9 in his body. If, however, your sport lies exclusively in the thick woodlands, or where only very long shots are likely to be had, supply yourself with numbers 2 or 3; but at the same time take care to provide a long and heavy gun, that will throw them even, and not in lumps and clusters.

PERCUSSION CAPS.—Detonating guns have now been so long in general use, that the familiarity thus produced with the various properties and kinds of fulminating powders, ensures the very general perfection to which these invaluable auxiliaries of the shooter have attained. They are to be had, of an almost uniform excellence, at all the respectable gunmakers in town and country.

WADDING.—Here again is a matter on which you will find a vast variety of opinion. Some get rid of it altogether by adopting the new system of cartridges. Upon this point I do not wish to offer any of the results of my own limited experience. I have shot with these, and with average success—a low average I admit, for I have no pretensions to the name of a crack. They are, however, worth the experiment of a trial, though I am disposed to believe the success or failure of it will much depend upon the accidental properties and effects of the materials submitted to the test. To return to the sort of wadding which may best serve those who still adhere to the old system of mere powder and shot. After enumerating the various claims of paper, hat, card, and leather, Colonel Hawker gives the preference to punched pasteboard,—the thickness to increase in the ratio of the diameter of the barrel. The best that have ever come under my notice are Cherry's prepared waddings, suited to every calibre. They are manufactured from felt which has undergone a process that prevents the accumulation of damp after firing, and are to be procured at any gunmaker's for the cost of the materials in ordinary use. These I do recommend, and I am sure those who accord them a trial will have no reason to regret it. They cover the powder effectually, and offer but little resistance to the shot, which is all that is required of wadding. **Mr.** Cherry would improve upon his invention by piercing the waddings intended to cover the shot, as it would facilitate the operation of loading, while the shooter made the distinction by carrying those for the powder in his left-hand pocket, and those for the shot in his right.

THE POWDER-FLASK.—It is strange that, among the many ingenious improvements effected in the implements of the shooter, the powder-flask, certainly the most important of all, should have been left in its present dangerous condition. I am aware that an attempt, and a praise-worthy one, was made some years ago by Mr. Egg, to reduce the chances of accident which the present construction of the flask involves; but I ask why has not some contrivance, without any of the old leaven in it, been suggested and effected? In the shot-belt the charger is wholly detached, where no risk, at all events, would follow, were it otherwise—whereas, when loading with powder, the charger, with the flask attached, is introduced into the muzzle of the gun, so that should it, by any accident, become ignited, an explosion (and most probably a fatal one) of the whole ensues as a matter of consequence. However, to deal with it as you find it, with proper precaution, when you fill your charger let back the spring gradually, that no chance may be given away in the event of a bit of flint, or any substance that might throw out a spark, being struck by it. Never lose sight of the material which your flask contains. Let nothing induce you to fire with it in your hand. If a chance shot offer while you are loading a discharged barrel, throw it behind you, if there is not time to return it to your pocket.

LOADING.—I have not thought it necessary to occupy any of my limited space with the shot-belt, because it is so

27

simple, and at the same time so excellent in construction, that the merest novice cannot be astray in the use of it. Not so is it with the important office—that of loading your gun aright, although it is impossible to lay down any rules for it applicable to every case. Experience alone will enable you so to proportion your charge that you shall come at the full powers of which your gun is capable. The gauge, the length, the weight—all must be taken into account, and provided for. For the ordinary run of fowling-pieces, the following is a fair proportion :—A shot-charger that holds an ounce and a half of shot may be filled to the brim with powder, which will serve to load with, as also to prime : the same measure filled up with shot will constitute your charge of lead. By these proportions, you can thus regulate the chargers of your belts and flasks. Against this system it is contended, by the ultra-particular, that it is a bad one in reference to powder, which is manufactured without regard to weight, only the projectile force being considered. These are minutiæ, however, into which I do not desire to introduce the learner. He will have enough to do with the more immediate affairs of preparing his nerves, forming a judgment upon sight and distance, and laying a foundation upon a basis of right principle and prompt performance, without which he will have little business upon that arena to which I am about to introduce him, after a long but still a necessary preface.

SHOOTING. THE FIELD.—Unless where some positive mental or physical prohibition exists, a certain degree of excellence and dexterity in every art and science is open to such as seek with care and perseverance. Thus, although, from natural causes, every man cannot aspire to the honor of becoming a crack shot, there is scarcely any that may not acquire the art of shooting tolerably well. The sooner the essay is made, the better the chance of its success; and as my pupil is supposed to be in this condition, I proceed, without further introduction, to offer such practical rules and maxims as may best serve to promote the end he should have in view—that of becoming cautious in the management, and steady in the use of his gun.

The first step, assuming the learner to be a complete novice, will be to acquire the proper mode of putting his gun to his shoulder, and of bringing the sight to bear upon a particular object,—the latter only to be rightly accomplished with the breech and sight on a level. Having attained this preliminary, let him take a flint gun, with a piece of wood substituted for the flint, and practise at the object so situated, always remembering to pull the trigger the moment the sight is on the mark—a precaution he will find the vast advantage of as he comes to apply it to flying shots. After a practise so conducted till the eye ceases to flinch when the trigger is drawn, he may begin to load with half charges, and continue to practise at his object, occasionally, without his knowledge, small charges of shot being added, so that he shall strike his mark without the nervous excitement of feeling that he is making the attempt.

The great point—that of steadiness combined with self confidence—being arrived at, he may now try his hand at small birds; but even after he has become adroit at these, he has still another ordeal to go through. This is the tremor at the springing of game, whether a pack of grouse, a covey of partridges, or a solitary cock-pheasant, which, indeed, often makes as startling a flight as either. In this case, it will serve him greatly to return to the system he began with, and learn to cover his game without the nervous apprehension of a miss. While at this practice, he may begin to use himself to cover with both eyes open, the advantage of which he will soon discover when he comes to quick shooting.

Being tolerably *au fait* at these points of practice (for perfection can only result from long experience, whence come skill and judgment), it will be necessary that he bear in mind those rules for rightly effecting his purpose when his game is moving. He must shoot before an object that crosses his point of sight; high for a bird rising in its flight, or skimming the surface; between the ears of hares or rabbits running in a straight line from him,—being guided, of course, in every case, by the distance between him and the mark at which he aims. For example, if a bird range forty yards from him, calculating the ordinary velocity of its speed of wing, he may safely aim six inches before it. No fixed rules, however, can be laid down, where the casualities of powder, a dull or lively shooting gun, and high winds, and fifty other et ceteras, are opposed to a system. One principle he may always adopt with success, and that is, to fix his eyes on the mark he has selected, and fire *the instant* the gun is brought to bear upon it. It is very difficult to say at what distance a bird may be which can be called a fair shot, because it rests with so many contingencies. Forty yards are generally considered as point-blank range, but it will often be found easier to bring down game at fifty than at thirty yards. The wind, as in cross shots, and various operating causes— all the result of temporary accident—must be taken into account. You will always have a better chance to kill long cross shots than those approaching or flying from you. It is very hard to do execution upon birds with a stern-chaser, and in coming towards you they present a surface off which shot is very apt to glance without penetrating. I have said nothing about the hold of his gun most convenient for the learner to accustom himself to, because, in whatever manner it may be put into his hands at first, he is sure, ultimately, to adopt a style of his own, arising from natural causes, or habits almost as forcible. The nearer it is placed to the guard, the less risk is run should a barrel burst. The grasp of the stock more forward affords the greatest facility in bringing the gun to bear upon its object, and more firmness of position.

While I am on the mechanical portion of the young shooter's acquirements, or rather things to be acquired, I do not think a better opportunity can be chosen to introduce a few hints upon a more advanced state of practice, albeit some may, at the time of perusing them, be unfit to receive what may be termed finishing lessons. When you are about taking a cross shot at a long range, fire well before it, from one to three feet, according to the speed with which the bird is flying, and let your gun be thrown above the object. The same rule must direct you in firing at hares or rabbits, whether it be a cross shot or one in a right line. It is a most mischievous practice, as far as regards your day's sport, to make much noise in the field, however strong the provocation from the disobedience of your dogs, or any cause whatever. Should your pointers prove incorrigible, I would rather recommend you, when they have sprung a covey, to cause them to be taken up, and then walk yourself as near as you can to the spot where you saw it drop. Should the birds rise singly or by the brace, continue to beat and shoot while you think one remains: it will be time enough to look after the slain (that cannot abscond) when you make sure of the living. This plan may also be successfully adopted when there is not scent enough to prevent the staunchest dogs from running in upon their game. In marking your covey

down, remember they cannot fall so long as they continue
to skim : they cannot alight till they stop themselves, and
prepare for the pitch, by a flapping of the wings.

I should not advise you to begin beating for partridges,
even in September, before nine o'clock, and then desist
from it at noon. From three till dusk is the golden division
of the day, at that season, for the partridge-shooter. If
your ground happen to lie in the vicinity of manors that
have been shot over during the day, you will be certain to
meet the remnants of scattered coveys, of all chances the
most sure to fill your game-bag. With pheasants, however,
when they are to be sought in strong covers, particularly,
your system must be almost reversed. As the day advances,
these birds resort to the thickest and strongest lying that
the woodlands frequented by them afford. When beating,
in the early morning, after rain, you will generally find
them in the skirts of covers, or in the hedgerows adjacent.
In such cases, always contrive to place yourself between
them and the strong old woods: to these they are certain
to fly,—instinct teaching them that there they are most
sheltered and secure. In *battue* shooting, all you have to
attend to is the situation of the best opens, and such sides
of the covers intended to be beaten, as the direction of the
wind, and the ordinary resort of the game, point out as the
most judicious stations ; but when about to engage in a
single-handed day's sport, you will require a more skillful
disposition, and closer attention to the manner of your
tactics. In this latter case, your best assistant will be a
steady old pointer ; one that will range near you, work
round every piece of copse and underwood, and poke into
every nook and crevice; well broke he must be, so as to
fall at shot, and crouch down on bringing in his birds.

In a treatise such as this, it would be impossible to give

even the briefest epitome of directions for the various
classes of game and wild-fowl shooting. Before, however,
I close my address to the young disciple of the trigger, I
will offer him a few familiar hints on a division of his craft
neither the least in importance or interest,—namely, his
relation to his best ally and friend, the dog. I am not
going to suggest the species best suited to general shooting,
as so very much depends upon the country to be hunted,
and the chance that may direct selection; but whether
pointer, setter, or spaniel, you will find your account in
making such as you intend for coadjutors in the field your
ordinary associates and companions. Try the experiment
by committing one puppy of a litter entirely to the breaker,
and retaining another (when the general rudiments of his
education have been acquired) constantly with yourself,
and at every opportunity subjected to gentle but firm discipline, and you will soon discover which is the better plan.
Adopt the same system with a perfectly made hunter—a
master of his business; and you will soon find out the
difference of being served by one who, from habit, will be
enabled to understand your looks, and another who, at best,
will have to puzzle out your wishes, or require to have them
announced at the hazard of flushing half the game in the
parish.

  With this parting word on the social economy of shooting,
closes the last of those notices of our FIELD SPORTS which
the publisher thought it convenient to appear in this
volume, and the treatment of which he confided to me. If
his purpose has been fulfilled, my desire will be accomplished,—the wish to please being our unity of design.
The little talent the writer possesses, at all events will not
have failed from lack of anxiety to accomplish his task :
what is writ is writ,—

"Would it were worthier!"

INDEX.

CHAMBERS' PAPERS FOR THE PEOPLE.

NOW COMPLETE IN 12 VOLUMES.

Fancy Colored Boards; also, bound in Six Volumes Cloth, Gilt, half Calf and Morocco, &c.,

100,000 COPIES SOLD IN ENGLAND!!

PUBLISHED BY

J. W. MOORE,

PUBLISHER, BOOKSELLER AND IMPORTER,

195 CHESTNUT STREET,

(Opposite the State House,)

PHILADELPHIA.

The **AMERICAN** is the fac simile of the English Edition, and is superior, inasmuch as full credit is given to **AMERICAN AUTHORS**.

This series is mainly addressed to that numerous class whose minds have been educated by the improved schooling, and the popular lectures and publications, of the last twenty years, and who may now be presumed to crave a higher kind of Literature than can be obtained through the existing cheap periodicals.

CONTENTS OF VOLUMES.

*

NOTICES OF THE PRESS.

TAYLOR'S STATISTICS OF COAL: Including Mineral Bituminous Substances employed in Arts and Manufactures; with their Geographical, Geological, and Commercial Distribution, and Amount of Production and Consumption on the American Continent; with Incidental Statistics of the Iron Manufacture. By R. C. Taylor, F. G. S. L., &c., &c. Second Edition, revised and brought down to 1854 by S. S. Haldeman, Prof. of Natural Science, &c. 1 vol. 8vo., colored maps and plates, $5.00.

[From the Scientific American.]

A new edition of Taylor's Statistics of Coal is published by J. W. Moore, of Philadelphia. When the first edition was published a few years ago, its thorough scientific character and accurate information at once brought new laurels to its able author. The *Edinburgh Review* passed a high eulogium upon it, and with no part of it have we ever heard a fault mentioned. This edition is revised and brought down to 1854, by Professor S. S. Haldeman, the venerable author having departed this life in 1851. It is chiefly devoted to the Coal and Iron natural resources of America; and no American, we assert, can have a proper idea of the vast internal resources of his country and be ignorant of the contents of this book. No library, public or private, can be complete without a copy of it. The publisher has spared no pains in making this an attractive work, it being embellished with numerous wood cuts and colored maps, printed on fine paper. 640 pages 8vo.

BURTON'S ANATOMY OF MELANCHOLY. What it is, with all the Kinds, Causes, Symptoms, Prognostics, and Several Cures of it. In Three Partitions; with their several Sections, Members, and Sub-sections, Philosophically, Medically, and Historically opened and cut up. A new edition, corrected and enriched by translations of the numerous classical extracts. To which is prefixed an account of the author. From the last London edition. 1 vol. 8vo., cloth, $2.50.

[*City Item.*]

The book is an inexhaustible fountain, where every mind, no matter what may be its peculiar organization, or the nature of its momentary needs, can draw at will nourishment and strength; such perfect mingling of immense erudition, profound thought, sparkling humor, and exuberant fancy, exists no where else out of Shakspeare.

THE WORKS OF MICHAEL DE MONTAIGNE, comprising his Essays, Letters, a Journey through Germany and Italy; with notes from all the Commentators, Biographical and Bibliographical Notices, &c., &c., &c. By William Hazlett. 1 vol. 8vo., pp. 686, cloth, $2.50.

[*Inquirer.*]

This is a truly valuable publication, and embodies much that may be read with profit.

[*North American.*]

This work is too well known, and too highly appreciated by the literary world, to require eulogy.

[*Hallam.*]

So long as an unaffected style and good nature shall charm —so long as the lovers of desultory and cheerful conversation shall be more numerous than those who prefer a lecture or a sermon—so long as reading is sought by the many as an amusement in idleness, or a resource in pain—so long will Montaigne be among the favorite authors of mankind.

THE KORAN, commonly called the Alcoran of Mahommed; translated into English immediately

from the original Arabic, with Explanatory Notes, taken from the most approved Commentators. To which is prefixed a preliminary discourse by George Sale, gent. A new edition, with a Memoir of the Translator, and with various readings and illustrative notes from Savary's Version of the Koran. 1 vol. 8vo., cloth. Numerous maps and plates, $2.50.

[*Louisville Journal.*]

This work is too well known to require a lengthy eulogy, and no library, public or private, is complete without this celebrated and interesting work. The publisher has spared no pains to make this an attractive work, being the sixth edition, printed on fine paper with numerous maps.

KNAPP'S LECTURES ON CHRISTIAN THEO-LOGY. Translated by Leonard Wood, Jun., D. D., President of Boudoin College, Brunswick, Maine. Sixth American Edition, $2.50.

This work is used as a Text Book in many of the Theological Schools of the United States.

THE COMPLETE PROSE WORKS OF JOHN MILTON, with a Biographical Introduction by Rufus W. Griswold. Bound in 2 vols. 8vo., and also one thick 8vo. vol.

This is the only edition of the complete prose works of that highly celebrated author, John Milton, that is published in this country, and it is needless to add that a copy should be found in every gentleman's library, and no public institution should be without a copy.

THE THEORY OF EFFECT, embracing the contrast of Light and Shade, of Color and Harmony.

By an Artist. With fifteen illustrations, by Hinckley. 18mo. cloth, 75 cents.

From the Baltimore Advertiser.

This work is by an artist of Philadelphia, and is an elementary treatise which will be found very useful so those who desire to learn the principles of the art of drawing. The work, though brief, contains many useful hints and suggestions of a practical character, together with simple and efficient rules.

THE CALCULATOR'S CONSTANT COMPANION for Practical Men, Machinists, Mechanics, and Engineers. By Oliver Byrne. $1.00.

From the Boston Daily Atlas.

This little volume is well adapted to its object, which is to be a labor-saving machine to practical men in making the necessary calculations of their daily business avocations, and will be found highly useful for all kinds of mechanics and engineers.

A MANUAL FOR PRACTICAL SURVEYS, containing methods indispensably necessary for Actual Field Operations. By E. W. Beans, Norristown, Montgomery Co., Pa. 18mo. cloth, 75 cents; 18mo. sheep, 75 cents; 18mo. tucks, $1.25.

From the London Artizan.

The author of this work is perfectly right when he says in his Preface, that "many of the publications in general use appear to have been written by those who were engaged in the instruction of youth, and who were unacquainted with the practical part of surveying." "There seems to be wanted a more minute detail of expedients employed in the field." This little work, which is not too bulky for the pocket, is just the sort of thing which a young surveyor ought to study before commencing practice; or he will find that all his fine problems, learned at school, will be thrown at his head by his impatient "chief." We therefore take pleasure in recommending this work.

THE INSTRUCTIVE GIFT; or, Narratives for the Young. Translated from the German. Illustrated by 8 beautiful colored plates. Cloth, $1.00; cloth, gilt, $1.25.

MY PLAY IS STUDY: A book for Children. Translated from the German by L. Lermont. Illustrated by 4 beautiful colored plates. Cloth, 62 cents; cloth, gilt, 75 cents.

EXAMPLES OF GOODNESS. Narrated for the Young. Translated for the Young. Translated from the German. Illustrated by 4 beautiful colored plates. Cloth, 62 cents; cloth, gilt, 75 cents.

ELLEN SEYMOUR; or, "The Bud and the Flower." By Mrs. Savile Shepherd, (formerly Miss Houlditch,) author of "Hymns adapted to the comprehension of Young Minds." 1 vol. 12mo. cloth, 88 cents; cloth, gilt extra, $1.25.

QUAKERISM; or, the Story of My Life. By a Lady who was for forty years a member of the Society of Friends. 12mo. cloth, $1.00.

CHAMBERS' INFORMATION FOR THE PEOPLE. A popular Cyclopedia, Tenth American Edition, with numerous additions, and more than five hundred Engravings. 2 vols. Royal 8vo. half morocco, $5.00.

CHAMBERS' REPOSITORY of Instructive and

Amusing Tracts, a Collection of choice Miscellaneous matter. Vols. 1 and 2 now ready. Fancy boards, 38 cents; cloth, 50 cents.

CHAMBERS' MISCELLANY of useful and entertaining Tracts, complete in 20 vols. Fancy boards, 38 cents; 10 vols. cloth, $7.50; 10 vols. half calf and morocco, $12.00.

AN EXPOSITION OF THE PROPHECIES OF THE APOCALYPSE, by the Rev. James De Pui, A. M., Chaplain in the United States Army. (Just published.) 12mo. cloth, 75 cents.

SMITH'S JUVENILE DRAWING BOOK, containing the rudiments of the Art, in a series of Progressive Lessons, 24 plates of subjects, easily copied. Small 4to. cloth, 16th edition, 75 cents.

HOUSEHOLD VERSES, by Bernard Barton. Embellished with a Vignette Title-Page and Frontispiece. 12mo. Illuminated covers. New edition, 50 cents. Cloth gilt, 75 cents.

COMMERCE OF THE PRAIRIES, or, The Journal of a Santa-Fe Trader, during eight expeditions across the Great Western Prairies, and a residence of nearly nine years in Northern Mexico. Illustrated with Maps and Engravings. By Josiah Gregg. 2 vols. 12mo., cloth $2.

MYSTERIES OF CITY LIFE; or, Stray Leaves

from the World's Book. By James Rees, author
of "The Philadelphia Locksmith," "The Night-
Hawk Papers," &c. 12mo. Paper, 75 cents.
Cloth, $1.

CHRISTIANITY, AND ITS RELATIONS TO
POETRY AND PHILOSOPHY, 12mo. Cloth,
50 cents.

AN AUTO-BIOGRAPHY AND LETTERS OF
CAROLINE FRY, the author of "The Listener,"
"Christ our Law," &c. 12mo., cloth, 75 cents.

WEEK AT GLENVILLE, by a Philadelphia Lady.
With numerous illustrations. Cloth, plain plates,
62 cents. Colored, 75 cents. Gilt edge, plain
plates, 75 cents. Colored, 88 cents.

BIBLIA HEBRAICA. Secundom Epitiones. Jos.
Athiae, Joannis Leusden, Jo. Simonis, Alirumque,
inprimis, Everardi Van Der Hooght, D. Henrici
Opitii, et Wolfii Heidin heim, cum additionibus
Clavique Masoretica et Rabbinica, Augusti Hahn.
Mune denuo recognita et emendata ab Isaaco
Leeser, V. D. M. et Josepho Jaquett, V. D. M.
The above is stereotyped from the last Leipsic
edition, and beautifully half bound in the German
style, thick 8vo. $3.

THE YOUNG MAN'S WAY TO HONOR, RE-
SPECTABILITY, AND USEFULNESS. By
Rev. Anthony Atwood. 18mo., cloth, 38 cents.
Gilt extra, 63 cents.

"A book that ought to be in the hands of every youth."